What
Really
Works

The Insider's Guide
to Natural Health

Susan Clark

Thorsons

While the author of this work has made every effort to ensure that the information contained in this book is as accurate and up to date as possible at the time of publication, medical and pharmaceutical knowledge is constantly changing and the application of it to particular circumstances depends on many factors. Therefore it is recommended that readers always consult a qualified medical specialist for individual advice. This book should not be used as an alternative to seeking specialist medical advice, which should be sought before any action is taken. The author and publishers cannot be held responsible for any errors or omissions that may be found in the text, or any actions that may be taken by a reader as a result of any reliance on the information contained in the text, which is taken entirely at the reader's own risk.

Thorsons
An Imprint of HarperCollins*Publishers*
77-85 Fulham Palace Road
Hammersmith, London W6 8JB

Published by Thorsons 2000

3 5 7 9 10 8 6 4 2

© Susan Clark 2000

Susan Clark asserts the moral right
to be identified as the author of this work

A catalogue record for this book
is available from the British Library

ISBN 0 7225 4026 4

Printed in Great Britain by Scotprint

For my mother, Anne

Let your mind run deep;
Let benevolence flood your relationships;
Let your words sing freely and true;
Let your decisions be peaceful and just;
Let your business be done well;
Let your actions be timely, fulling and complete.

Lao Tzu

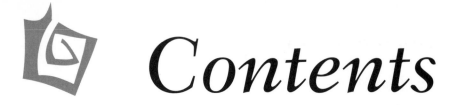

Contents

Acknowledgements

With special thanks to
Dr Peter Mansfield and Max Tomlinson for all their assistance, especially reading this manuscript.

With thanks for their help, support and guidance:
My husband, Declan O'Mahony, my sister, Melissa Clark and my co-author Erick Muzard, my agent Teresa Chris, my VA Carol Golcher, researcher Julia Donovan, my editor at Thorsons/HarperCollins, Wanda Whiteley, Jeremy Langmead, former editor of *The Sunday Times'* Style magazine Penny Wark, deputy features editor of *The* [London] *Times* Vicki Grimshaw and Keith Kendrick, editor of *Chat* magazine.

With special thanks for their inspiration to:
Jane Waters, Leslie Kenton, Wayne Dyer, Diana Cooper, Vera Taggart, Swamiji, Fidelma Spilsbury, Ceridwen.

With grateful thanks for their generosity in sharing their knowledge and in supporting my work:
Richard Allport, holistic veterinary practitioner, Ray Bailey, Julian Baker, the European College of Bowen Studies, Stephan Ball, author and Bach Flower Remedy practitioner, Belinda Barnes, Foresight (formerly The Association of Pre-Conceptual Care), Alick Bartholomew, The Kombucha Tea Network (UK), Dr Eliot Berson, Harvard University, Sanjay and Meenu Bhandari, Farmacia, Jonathan Brostoff, Professor of Allergy and Environmental Health, University College London Medical School, Deni Brown, The Herb Society, Jane Burton,

PR, Anthony Bush, Maurice Hanssen and Penny Viner, The Health Food Manufacturers Association (UK), Dr Etienne Callebout, complementary cancer specialist, Kitty Campion, herbalist and author, Drs Adam and Beverley Carey, co-founders of The Centre for Nutritional Medicine, Andrew Chevalier, herbalist, Dr James Colthurst, homeopath and KOSMED practitioner, Tina Cooke, founder of The Cancer Alternative Information Bureau, David Crawford, nutritionist and kinesiologist, Sue Croft, Consumers for Health, John Davidson, Wholistic Research Company and author, Dr Valerie Dias, The Integrated Health Partnership, Gaynor and Mike Donaldson, Hambleden Herbs, Michael Donovan, PR, Aidan and Micha Ellis, Ellis Organics, David and Margaret Evans, Robert Farago, hypnotherapist, Sandra Gibbons, co-founder and director of The Alternative Centre, Professor Glenn Gibson, Food Research Institute, Reading University, Dr Marilyn Glenville, author and nutritionist, Gilli Harouvi, Astanga yoga teacher, Tel Aviv, Israel, Colette Harris, *Here's Health*, Anthony and Bharti Haynes, nutrition consultants and co-founders of The Nutrition Clinic, Dr Robert Hempleman, holistic dental practitioner, Susie Hewson, Bodywise, Angela and John Hicks, founders and joint principals of The Integrated College of Chinese Medicine, Reading, UK – and both excellent practitioners, Patrick Holford, nutritionist, author and founder of The Institute of Optimum Nutrition, Dr Charles Innes, homeopath, Paddy Lane, National Retreat Association, Dr Jack Levenson, founder of the British Society for Mercury-Free Dentistry, Graham Lewis, Rio Trading Company, Dr George Lewith, consultant physician in complementary medicine and co-founder of The Centre for the Study of Complementary Medicine, Eleanor Lines, *The CompMed Bulletin*, Eric Llewelyn, founder of Nature's Own, Dr Andrew Lockie, homeopath and author, Alison Loftus, nutritionist, Roz Kadir, nutritionist, Dr Brian Kaplan, homeopath, Marie Kendal, Women into Complementary Health, Dr Julian Kenyon, co-founder of The Centre for the Study of Complementary Medicine, Alison

Kilmartin, Patients Against Mercury Amalgams, Dr Leonard McEwan, Michael McIntyre, herbalist and chairman of the European Herbal Association, Dr Gillian McKeith, nutritionist, Dr Deborah McManners, naturopath, Lynne McTaggart and Andrew Miller, *What Doctors Don't Tell You* monthly newsletter, Dr Peter Mansfield, director and founder of Good HealthKeeping, Ian Marber, nutritionist and author, Kathryn Marsden, nutritionist and author, Rohit Mehta, The Nutricentre, Graeme Miller, publisher and editor, *Journal of Alternative and Complementary Medicine*, Dian Mills, nutritionist, Jonathan Monckton, Research Council for Complementary Medicine, Charles Montagu, hypnotherapist and founder of The Health Partnership, Emma Moore, Health & Beauty Director, *The Sunday Times*, Tom Moses, *Country Life*, Diana Mossop, founder of Phytobiophysics, Robin Munro, Yoga Therapy Trust, Catherine O'Driscoll, founder of the Canine Defence League, Audrey Pasternak, practitioner of The Metamorphic Technique, Sue Pennington, yogi and inspirational teacher of Astanga and Iyengar yoga, Tony Pinkus, director of Ainsworths, the homeopathic pharmacy, Penelope Povey, medical herbalist, Lynne and Geoffrey Robinson, The Pilates Association, Andre Sanford, homeopath, Elizabeth Seasons, naturopath, Dr Rajendra Sharma, practitioner and author, Helen Sher, skin psychotherapist and founder of the Sher Skincare System, Charles Siddle, animal healer, Dr Fritz Smith, founder of Zero Balancing, Dr J Somper, homeopath, Maryon Stewart, author and founder of the Women's Nutritional Advisory Service, Michael van Straten, naturopath, author and broadcaster, Dr Padmini Tekur, University of Bombay, Stephen Terrass and Marie Kendal, Solgar Vitamins, Max Tomlinson, naturopath and author, Jacqueline Tuson, The Centre for the Study of Complementary Medicine, Charlotte Vontz, The Green People Company, Raj Vora, The Revital Health Shops, Bharti Vyas, holistic beauty therapist, Anne Walker, Department of Nutrition, Reading University, UK, Jane Waters, co-founder and director of

The Alternative Centre, author and practitioner, Zeta West, midwife and Traditional Chinese Medicine specialist, Christopher Whitehouse, Consumers for Health Choice, David Wilkie, Olympic Gold Medallist and founder of Health Perceptions, Celia and Brian Wright, Higher Nature.

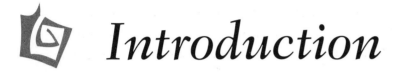 # *Introduction*

You know St John's Wort is nature's own Prozac and good for mild to moderate depression, but you don't know how much to take or for how long. You read somewhere that rotting banana skins can help heal a verruca, or was that one you imagined? Your sister told you there's a great new hands-on massage treatment which will leave you feeling revitalised and centred, but you've forgotten the name and you'd love to escape to one of the new 'spiritual spas', but don't know where to go or what to take with you.

If these are the kinds of things that race around your brain as you try to keep up with what's new in holistic and complementary health, then this is the book for you. If you're forever cutting health and lifestyle snippets from newspapers and magazines and then losing them, or if you push your trolley around the supermarket trying to remember which is better – oat bran or wheat bran? – then *What Really Works* has the answer.

Packed with cutting-edge advice and proven tips to help you lead a more holistic and nourishing life, it takes the legwork out of figuring out how best to enjoy optimum health and well-being for the rest of your life. You don't have to do the research because I've done it for you.

In the first section, BodyWorks, you will learn, for example, about the most important five building blocks of good health – Food, Air, Water, Sunlight and Exercise. You'll find out why prebiotics are the next big wave in digestive health and how to breathe properly again. Find out why you should not be hiding indoors from sun and how a form of Tai Chi with a broom handle (of all things!) can help keep you in good physical shape.

Section II, which is called Top-to-Toe, is an A–Z of everyday health complaints, from acne to vitiligo. Here you will find the same no-nonsense advice that has made my weekly columns in *The Sunday Times*, *The Times* and *The Sun* such a hit with 18 million readers. You'll discover it's true that a banana skin can help get rid of a verruca – but only if you tape the blackened inside of the skin over the head of the wart. You'll also learn why homocysteine, a normal byproduct of metabolism, is a more important indicator of potential heart problems than cholesterol, and find out how you can reverse lots of digestive disorders.

Again, I've read the books, interviewed the health gurus and been pummelled and prodded by a variety of hands-on therapists so that I can report back on *what really works*. You will find the best nutritional, herbal, homeopathic and other natural remedies to 80 conditions, ranging from whey protein concentrate for athlete's foot to nettle tea for the common and distressing Irritable Bowel Syndrome.

Section III, Hands-On, will help you sort your Reiki (pronounced ray-key) from your Metas (Metamorphic Technique). If you've never heard of either, this A–Z section will unravel the mystery and help you decide which complementary treatment best suits you, your stage in life or any particular problem you may currently have. We've reviewed some of the very best complementary therapies and can tell you how to find a good practitioner, what will happen during treatment, and what you will feel during the session and after.

Discover, too, how just two supplements and a common herb will give you the same energy levels you had 10 years ago and find out more about the new concept of energy and vibrational medicine, which encourages practitioners to treat the cause and not the symptoms of an illness.

In SoulWorks, we turn to spiritual health – every bit as important as your physical well-being. This section draws from the world's richest and most potent healing traditions to put you back in touch with your own inner voice. Find out how animals bring signs from those guiding you on your spiritual path. Discover the significance and the names of your own power animals, and learn some of the shamanic techniques that all our ancestors practised before modern medicine was born, when everyone accepted that sickness was a reflection of an ailing soul.

You will, and may already have, found you own spiritual path, but in the chapter devoted to Prayer & Meditation I will introduce you to a simple but powerful meditation technique where you get all the anti-stress and inner health benefits of stilling the mind, without having to sit on a cold, hard floor or remembering to chant '*om*'.

Finally, the last chapter, Time Out, shows you how to nourish your soul by taking off on a spiritual retreat. Forget limp lettuce leaves and carrot juice. The spiritual spa has taken over from the health farm as the ultimate escape for those seeking a new way of living. You can have warm oil poured over your mystical third eye, book an holistic body massage with a therapist who has trained for seven years with Thai monks or practise your yoga Sun Salutations to the sound of the Caribbean sea lapping the palm-fringed shore. In this chapter I recommend my own personal list of the Top 10 best secret hide-aways that really will give your mind, body and soul a break. You won't find these in any spa or guidebook but you will, if you go to any of them, return to your daily life feeling inspired and spiritually renewed.

One of the biggest criticisms of complementary treatments is that there is no true evidence to show they work. This is rubbish. You just have to dig for it. Of course, most people do not have time to scour the latest scientific papers, read every new health book or talk to the experts, but that is my job. I am never off duty and I love what I do. I consider myself lucky to get paid for it, and even more fortunate to be able to pass what I learn on so that other people can also take responsibility for their own health.

This is not a book you have to read from cover to cover but, if you like, a reference manual which you can dip in and out of at will. There's an excellent

Resources section to help you find the practitioners and products you need to stay healthy, and a comprehensive Bibliography to help you start to build your own 'health library', or simply find out more.

Throughout the writing of this book, I've had one vivid image in mind. I live in the Chiltern Hills in Oxfordshire, about an hour out of London and opposite a lush green beechwood. As the idea of a book which bridged my twin interests of complementary health and a more sacred way of living took root, I noticed that the early summer foxgloves outside my home were growing with renewed vigour.

One afternoon, while walking my dog, I strayed from the marked footpath and stumbled across a magnificent row of six-footers; standing like sentries guarding the woodland. I had never noticed foxgloves in that spot before and I don't know if I'll ever see them again, but what struck me was the realisation that each and every one had its roots firmly in the woodland soil and shade but was growing, as fast as it could, towards the light.

I can't think of a better metaphor for that new and more sacred way of living that so many of us have now set our hearts on. Take a detour from your own fixed path and you too will find yourself reaching away from the shadows towards the light. My wish for my book is that it will be a tool to help other like-minded people find the inner strength to recognise their own journey and embark on it.

Susan Clark
www.WhatReallyWorks.co.uk

BodyWorks

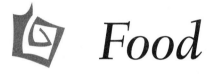 # *Food*

The Artificial Gut

In a humble laboratory at the Institute of Food Research in the UK, there is a machine which operates exactly like a real human gut. Each day, it is 'fed' different foods so that the scientists can figure out just what does go on in the human colon. What they are particularly interested in is the balance of the bacteria in the human gut. What, for example, happens to the bacteria which normally help us digest our food when the diet is too high in sugar? How does the artificial gut cope with antibiotics or prescription drugs, including the contraceptive pill? How does a gut that is fed infant formula differ from one that is nourished with human breastmilk, and what happens when the researchers deliberately change the gut flora by introducing man-made molecules that can ct as a kind of fast food for the good bacteria and which also work in the body to starve the toxic bad ones?

The work that is quietly going on in this lab is not to be laughed at or dismissed lightly, because if vitamin and mineral supplements were the first wave of getting back to good health in the 20th century, then the secrets of the human gut, which has to process these dietary supplements, holds the key to optimum health in this new century.

It is not right to say 'you are what you eat'. You are, though, a reflection of how your body *absorbs* what you eat, and for too many adults in the West, the honest answer when asked 'how are you?' is 'not great'.

This does not mean you are sick. You function. You get out of bed each day, run a household, sort out the kids, hold down a job, but you never feel 100%. You may be tired all the time, your skin may be less than glowing. Maybe you just don't have the energy to get out there and exercise. However it shows up, you know you could be better.

Digestive disorders are the root cause of 70% of all complaints and health problems, according to naturopaths who treat illness with a combination of nutrition, homeopathy and herbalism. Gut problems now cause more days off work (after the common cold) than any other health problem, and a third of the adult population is troubled by Irritable Bowel Syndrome (IBS), where the symptoms alternate between chronic constipation and diarrhoea.

More frightening is the fact that cancer of the colon is now the second biggest cancer killer after cancer of the breast in women and lung cancer in men. In humans, it is now believed that tumours arise 100 times more often in the large intestine, compared with the small one. What scientists must now find out is whether some of the large intestinal bacteria are actually producing carcinogenic or tumour-promoting compounds as a byproduct of their own metabolism. If this is what is going on, the solution may be as simple as changes to the diet.The progress of a colon cancer is slow, making it more than susceptible to the right kind of dietary intervention.

What to Eat

The message has not changed, so if you care about your health, you will have probably heard it before. If you want to avoid some of the worst toxins now used in the production of nutrient-poor foods from nutrient-robbed soils – and at the last count, there were an estimated 250,000 of them – switch to an organic diet wherever you can.

Organic food has been produced without the use of chemicals to protect the crop from insects or accelerate crop growth, and so while it may have been fashionable of late to join a backlash claiming there is no difference between organic and non-organic food, adopting this view flies in the face of both science and common sense.

Hard evidence that organic food is healthier to eat than conventional crops has now been published by scientists who claim they finally have the proof that plants grown without artificial pesticides and fertilisers contain higher levels of nutrients.

The study is one of the first to confirm what those of us who intuitively support organic farming have long suspected – that organic fruit and vegetables do not just taste better, but offer greater health benefits too.

Researchers backed by Britain's organic watchdog The Soil Association compared plants grown under strict organic conditions with those grown by conventional farming methods. The team, based at the University of Copenhagen, found that organic plants contained higher levels of vitamins and far more 'secondary metabolites' – a family of compounds which help protect plants from outside attack. When eaten in fresh fruit and vegetables, some of these metabolites are thought to lower the risk of cancer and heart disease.

There is no question too, that increasing the amount of raw food in your diet will also make you healthier. This is because a raw food diet will boost levels of the enzymes we need to break down and digest our food, at every stage of this process from the mouth to the gut. Even a short time on a mostly raw food diet can help detox the body, boost energy levels and help normalise the digestive tract. I have included three simple but powerful detox diets in this book (see pages 130, 136 and 147). Try them and watch how, as your health gets better on the inside, this is reflected on the outside as the condition of your skin, hair and nails improve beyond recognition.

For everyday eating, government guidelines in most countries suggest you aim for five portions of fruit and vegetables daily. For optimum health, though, you should actually be aiming for eight. Thankfully, that means eight in total – that is, fruit *or* veg, not eight of each.

People often get confused about what constitutes a portion. There is no need to fret about exact weights or to spend hours counting the broccoli florets in your raw vegetable side-salad, but as a rough guideline a portion is the equivalent of a slice of bread, half a bowl of rice, half a standard side-salad, a broccoli spear or a small apple.

Aiming for eight portions is easier said than done, of course, since most people hate chomping their way through what are laughingly called 'health foods'. Maybe not so funny, since, as this term implies, so many foods are not healthy at all. In fact, if you do give in to a junk diet and spend years eating these more popular but nutritionally-starved foods, then far from nourishing you, they will eventually make you sick.

If you are in any doubt that the food on your plate really can affect your health, reflect on this: in Japan, where the diet is rich in substances called phytochemicals, especially soya, 25% fewer women succumb to breast cancer than in the West. Men, too, benefit from these nutrients, because while the rates of prostate cancer in the East and the West are similar, far fewer Japanese men will actually die of the disease.

Conversely, cancer rates among East Asians who migrate and adopt Western diets mimic those of the Western world, within a shockingly short period of time.

Cheat Your Way to Better Health

Juicing is the ultimate cheat to better health. It's the quickest way to get live enzymes straight into the stomach and bloodstream, and is also the fast-track way to eat those eight portions of raw fruit and vegetables without getting jaw ache. Think about it: You need to juice about 16 medium-sized carrots to make a glass of carrot juice for breakfast. Despite the fact that carrots are a superb source of antioxidant compounds called monoterpenes and betacarotenes, which help protect against killer cancers and heart disease if eaten regularly, you probably don't eat half that number in a week.

Juicing used to be as dull as ditchwater, but there are now lots of excellent and inspiring new juicing books (see the Bibliography), so if, after a few weeks of juice therapy, you're still stuck with carrot and celery, you will only have yourself to blame.

You can juice, blend and pulp any vegetable, fruit or seed you care to name. Can't face grinding your way through a bowl of selenium-rich prostate-protecting brazil nuts? Make a nut milk instead. Nut milks are an excellent alternative to dairy, especially for kids who have allergies to milk but who can tolerate nuts. Since nuts are also rich in the essential fatty acids (especially omega-3s) which work in the body to dislodge stored fat, they can even help with weight loss and tackle unsightly cellulite.

You can buy a decent standard juicer for less than £50, but if you're serious about juicing or if you suffer from any of the digestive disorders detailed later in this book (see Top-to-Toe) and which mean you should be aiming for a 70% raw food diet, then The Champion Juicer is the one all the professionals use. It's actually quite sleek-looking and not too bad to clean. It can pulp, mash and grind, and while it is not cheap, it is a reliable workhorse that will not let you down.

Eat with the Seasons

Eating with the seasons not only means you are getting your food fresh, it also brings real health benefits. Fresh young spring greens, for example, help cleanse and detoxify your system after the stagnation of winter. Warm, nourishing root vegetables sustain the body through the colder months of winter, and in the summer, light salads and juicy ripe fruits will keep energy levels high and the body hydrated.

Why Are You Still Eating Meat?

At the risk of upsetting meat-producers everywhere, I have to report that whenever I analyse the nutrutional content of any meat recipe, I find it hard to justify its place in any health book ... including my *Vitality Cookbook!* Most meat contains cholesterol-raising hidden saturated fats and, unless you buy organic, it's quite likely to contain more than lingering traces of the antibiotics animals are pumped full of to promote faster growth and higher profit margins.

There are lots of reasons to stop eating meat. Buddhists and Hindus, for example, believe that when you eat meat you lower your spiritual vibrations, and that with every mouthful you swallow the terrifying death screams of the animal which at its slaughter, often at the hand of someone it trusted to feed and nurture it, seeps into the memory of the muscle tissues.

If that's too far out for you and you don't, in any event, object to meat on a soul level, then think about your physical health. Vegetarians are three times less likely to have a heart attack or a stroke than meat-eaters. They have a 40% lower incidence of cancer and are less likely to suffer from arthritis, obesity, diet-related diabetes, constipation, gallstones, hypertension and many other ailments.

If you don't care about your health, what about your figure? When did you last see a fat tree or a fat vegetarian? Neither of these depends on meat for survival, and nor do we. The inner lining of the human colon is pocketed to slow down digestion. This, according to nutritional anthropologists, suggests that our natural diet should be one of fruit and vegetables. The inner surface of the colon of a canine animal like the dog is smooth and unpocketed for fast transit and the digestion of meat.

Meat that stays in the gut rots in the gut and can cause additional problems including diverticulosis and bad breath. Think what a piece of meat would look and smell like if you left it on the worktop in the kitchen for four days. US researchers reckon that, on average, there's eight pounds of undigested, putrefying meat in the intestines of an adult American.

Still dying for that medium rare steak?

When and How to Eat

If you are eating the right foods – and, just as importantly, at the right times – you should be able to eat as much as you like, when you like. Digesting food, converting it to energy that the body can use and eliminating waste takes an astonishing 80% of your total energy reserves. No wonder, then, that so many people who have irregular mealtimes, impaired digestion and no time to prepare good food for themselves feel tired all the time – the amount of energy they are spending on the whole process must be even higher.

Smaller, more frequent meals make less of a demand on your digestive tract than one or two large and late-night meals. Adopt a 'nil by mouth' policy after 5 p.m., and any excess weight you carry will naturally drop off.

The French, of course, savour their meal times and you would never catch them wolfing their way through some gastronomic delight with eyes glued to the TV. The *way* we eat our food is just as important as *what* we eat, and the guidelines I like to follow, whenever possible, are those put forward by Ayurvedic practitioners, who take their inspiration from India. (For a full explanation of Ayurveda – or the ancient Indian 'science of life' – see page 272).

One simple but highly effective tip from these practitioners, especially for those of you suffering digestive disorders, is to make and drink a special ginger pickle 30 minutes before each meal. The pickle, a combination of honey, freshly grated root ginger and lemon juice, together with a pinch of salt, all dissolved in warm water, does not taste as bad as it sounds. In fact it has a warming quality and, I can promise you, it definitely works.

Other healthy eating tips from the older healing traditions include leaving the table when you are three-quarters full (this is customary in yoga traditions); replacing your cutlery on the plate between mouthfuls to slow the rate at which you eat, avoiding all gassy or fizzy drinks and taking a short walk to help ease digestion after each meal.

The most important thing is to make time for the food you have prepared, and that means setting the table and sitting down to eat. Even when you are alone. Eating on the hoof may be tempting when you are in a rush but you will, eventually, pay for this bad habit with a disruption to your digestion.

True Nutrition

Many humble, everyday foods bring huge health benefits. Did you know, for example, that rhubarb is an excellent source of calcium, or that eating just two apples a day can reduce blood cholesterol levels by 16%? True nutrition would have nothing to do with supplements and everything to do with what you choose to put on your plate.

The biggest irony in modern medicine is that doctors have little or no training in nutrition – in the UK, most qualify with just an hour of nutritional training – yet the very idea that good nutrition is paramount comes from their own founding father, Hippocrates who said: 'Let food be thy medicine' and who believed that adjusting the diet should be the first step in any treatment to alleviate or prevent ill health.

The following guidelines show just how easy it is for all of us to use food as medicine:

Beating Stress: The B vitamins are known as nature's own stress busters. They always work better together than when eaten alone, and are found in foods as diverse as bananas, cheese, sunflower seeds and soya. Eat lentils and brown rice for vitamin B_6, which can alleviate nausea and help treat morning sickness; eat dairy products and fish for B_{12}, which boosts energy and improves memory and concentration. Dark, leafy green vegetables are rich in folic acid, which can slow down ageing and help prevent heart problems.

Banishing Fatigue: Coenzyme Q10 (CoQ10) is an antioxidant vitamin-like substance needed to produce energy in every single cell in the body. Frequently taken by athletes to increase stamina, it bolsters the immune system and revitalises the body by boosting circulation, increasing the oxygenation of tissues and strengthening muscles. Food sources include tuna, spinach, sardines, peanuts, mackerel, sesame seeds and legumes, but it is highly perishable and easily destroyed by cooking, storing and processing, so eat as many of these foods raw – say in the form of Japanese sushi – as you can. Magnesium also plays a crucial role in the production of energy – eat fish, seafood, green leafy vegetables, whole grains, nuts, lemons, figs, apples, apricots, bananas and brown rice.

Boosting Immunity: High cholesterol levels can prevent white blood cells from getting to infected sites and from multiplying, so keep the saturated fat content of your diet down and watch out for hidden fats in processed foods and meats. Disease-fighting white blood cells are also slower to mobilise after alcohol consumption, so cut back on drinking. Vitamin A promotes thymus health, which in turn supports the immune system, so eat lots of yellow fruits and vegetables, organic dairy products and oily fish. Vitamin C is also a potent immune booster: eat citrus fruits, broccoli, kale, peas, tomatoes, orange juice, kiwi fruits, guava and papaya. Shiitake and Reishi mushrooms are also used as immune enhancers in Asian food.

Balancing Hormones: Hormones serve as the body's messengers. They are secreted into the bloodstream by different organs, and different hormones have specific jobs. Even minor fluctuations in hormone levels can have a dramatic impact on the body. Thanks to the use of synthetic hormones in medicine and xeno-oestrogens in the environment and food production, our hormones have never been under greater threat. Phytochemicals, derived from natural plant substances such as soya, help rebalance hormones that have gone haywire. They act as adaptogens, preventing, for example, too much oestrogen from locking on to receptor sites in the body, and, conversely, boosting levels when they fall lower than normal. Foods containing these substances include soya, citrus fruits, vegetables, cereals, onions, garlic, broccoli, cabbage and cauliflower.

Boosting Brainpower: Folic acid is crucial for proper brain function, yet surveys show it is one of the nutrients most deficient in our diets. Food sources include spinach, asparagus, turnip, greens, root vegetables, brewer's yeast and brussels sprouts. Vitamin B_{12} improves memory and concentration. Cheese, eggs, fish, clams and dairy products are all good sources. The amino acid Lysine will also boost brain power. Eat fish, soya products, cheese, yeast and lima beans when you need to be sharp and alert.

Aiding Digestion: Magnesium is crucial for proper bowel function, but is the second most common mineral deficiency in both sexes. Good natural sources include seafood, whole grains, dark leafy green vegetables and nuts. Add fibre-rich ground psyllium seeds to your food; avoid mucus-forming dairy products and keep caffeine down to a minimum.

Elimination is as important as digestion; the best way to flush toxins from the body is to drink a cup of warm water and lemon juice every morning and to fast one day a week. The herb Pau d'arco will also help restore the pH balance of the colon and promote healing. It tastes very planty but has excellent detoxifying properties, so make it an acquired taste. Bananas also help repopulate the good bacteria in the gut, which aid digestion – so make lots of banana smoothies.

Revitalising Your Skin: Intestinal health is crucial for glowing skin, so follow all the above to help regulate the bowels and keep the colon healthy. The skin is not just the body's protective wrapping – it's your largest organ too. Vitamin A is important for its maintenance, so eat lots of those yellow fruits and vegetables which are rich in carotenoids. Zinc, which is plentiful in oysters, pumpkin seeds, herring, eggs, crabmeat, turkey and seafood, will also help. Eat broccoli, tofu, green leafy vegetables and organic dairy produce too.

Revving Up Your Sex Life: Most people are surprised to learn that nutrition plays any role at all in sexual function and performance, but the sex hormones are controlled by the glands of the endocrine system, all of which can themselves be specifically nourished by certain nutrients. The B vitamins, for example, enter the cells of the thyroid gland to act as energisers and increase the hormonal flow. One way to boost the hormones responsible for libido is to mix 2 tablespoons of Brewer's yeast with 2 tablespoons of wheat germ in a glass of organic vegetable juice. Drink this with your evening meal and the nutrients will be assimilated by bedtime.

The pituitary gland controls the sex hormones, and needs vitamin E and zinc, as well as the B vitamins, to function at optimum levels. Eat the same foods as above for zinc, and peanuts, almonds, pecans and brazil nuts for vitamin E.

Functional Foods

Back to that laboratory at the UK's Institute of Food Research, where one of the most exciting projects being pioneered is the development of prebiotics. Many people have now heard of probiotics – foods or supplements which replenish levels of good bacteria in the gut – but prebiotics are an even more clever and natural concept. They take the biochemical process a stage back from probiotics.

What prebiotics do is work to rebuild the remaining levels of good bacteria by feeding them up to make them strong and dominant again. (See Fructo-oligosaccharides, known as FOS, page 100). As with probiotics, which are now common in yoghurts and other health drinks, prebiotics can easily be incorporated into everyday foods such as biscuits and breakfast cereals.

But among the more ingenious ideas currently being researched by Professor of Microbiology Glenn Gibson and his team is that of a 'designer' prebiotic which is combined with free-floating receptor chemicals that attract and then bind the toxic and possible cancer-causing bacteria strains. This would stop them from binding to the gut wall and, instead, flush them swiftly out of the colon before they can cause any serious or irreversible damage.

Professor Gibson, who co-built the first artificial colon in the UK, says:

It takes, on average, 70 hours for residual foodstuffs to pass through the colon where several hundred different species of bacteria are present. One important development and our real challenge now is that of synbiotics – where prebiotics and probiotics are combined in the same supplement.

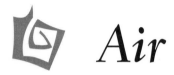 *Air*

> **Deprive the body of oxygen and, within minutes, you will die. Without the breath, there is no life.**

If you weren't breathing you'd be dead. Right? Of course. So why do you need to read anything about how to breathe? A newborn baby can do it without a self-help manual, so why devote an entire chapter of a book to something that should be so instinctive?

The reason is that somewhere between that first gasp of oxygen into our tiny infant lungs, growing up and becoming adults who barely have time to catch their breath between one task and the next, most of us have forgotten how to breathe properly.

During an average day, you will take 12 breaths a minute. That adds up to 17,280 breaths each and every day of your life. In a healthy person, the diagphragm is responsible for up to 70% of respiration, leaving the rest to the chest and other respiratory muscles. That means, if I ask you to take a deep breath and you puff out your chest, you are not breathing as nature intended, using the full and generous capacity of your lungs which, if spread over a flat surface, would cover an area roughly the size of a tennis court.

One theory which tries to explain the growing number of degenerative diseases people suffer in the West is that many of them are caused by insufficient oxygen reaching the body's tissues and organs. In recent years, cosmetic and alternative therapies based on oxygen-therapies have mushroomed.

If you stop, right now, and simply become aware of your own breathing you will see how just by paying attention to something you normally do subconsciously, it automatically changes. Once you start to concentrate on your breath, it will probably slow down, which is what happens in deep relaxation and meditation. You may have a strong urge to sigh and release a build-up of tension that you have now only just become aware of, even though it has been there throughout the time you have been reading this.

Let go of this deep sigh but keep your mouth closed so that the air escapes down through the nose. Lots of people teach breathing techniques where you breathe in through the nose and out through the mouth. In yoga, which is where I re-learned how to breathe properly, we never let air in or out through the mouth but always rely on the nose, which has special filters or *microvillae* (minute hairs) to filter out pollutants and prevent the worst of them from getting into the lungs. It also means the air must travel further to reach the lungs and so gives it the chance to warm up to body temperature and humidity en route.

The fact is, we pay scant regard to our pattern of breathing throughout our normal daily activities, and it is only when someone brings it to our attention that we realise many of us 'shallow breathe' our way through life most of the time. Try to take that deeper breath and the chances are your shoulders will rise, you will puff out your chest and draw the air from somewhere in the region of the back of your throat.

This is because you are only using the upper regions of the lungs. What you should be doing is breathing in from the diaphragm. Unless you are a musician, you probably won't know where this is, let alone how to use it, and because of this you will probably be using less than a third of your entire lung capacity.

Learning how to breathe properly again not only helps calm and quieten the mind but has also been shown to strengthen the immune system and improve the cardiovascular supply so that more oxygen is delivered around the body. People who run regularly, and so breathe deeply, also suffer all the usual age-related complaints at a much slower rate than non-runners.

Healthy lungs use only 3% of the body's total energy. Diseased lungs will suck up more than a third of your energy reserves. Thankfully, learning to breathe properly is both enjoyable, since it is so soothing, and easy. As well as nourishing all our body's tissues and fuelling its different systems, air keeps the mind sharp. The brain uses three times more oxygen than other organs, so if you are feeling sluggish, get breathing.

How to Breathe

A true breath starts by expanding the muscles of the diaphragm down and out.
Then pushes them up and in again. This enables the lungs to expand to their full
capacity, allows air to rush into them and helps it to be vigorously expelled.
Breathing this way, even for a short while, is very re-energising.

Few forms of Western exercise attach any importance at all to how you breathe,
but in yoga the breath and a rhythmic pattern of breathing is so important that a
whole discipline is devoted to it: Pranayama. *Prana* means life and *yama* means
its cessation.

The average volume of air you take in with a single breath is about 328 cubic
centimetres. This can vary, of course, depending on your size, sex, posture,
emotional and physical state and your environment. What the pranayama yogi
teachers believe is that by re-learning how to breathe, you can increase this
volume to 1640 cubic centimetres – a five-fold rise.

The lung tissues grow less elastic with age, but deep yogic breathing can reverse
this deterioration and boost the body's overall metabolism. It is so effective that
there are now specialised Pranic healers who do nothing but teach the value of
proper breathing to cleanse and strengthen the physical and spiritual body. The
yogis believe that prana is a special, almost spiritual force which circulates with
the oxygen and which travels through the body via a series of complex energy
channels called the *nadis*. These are similar, in pattern, to our physical nerves
and blood vessels but are governed by the chakras (see Chapter 10).

Yogic Breathing

In yoga, practitioners say that where the breath is, you'll find the mind. What they mean is that if you can begin to control the breath, you can also begin to marshall the mind and free it from the stresses and strains of everyday life and its demands.

One of my favourite breathing exercises comes from the Sivananda discipline, one of the yoga schools which treat prana – the breath of life – with as much, if not more respect as the asanas or positions which are also practised to tone the body, cleanse the mind and massage the internal organs.

One of the simplest of these is called *Anuloma Viloma*, or alternate nostril breathing. It is very calming and helps rebalance energy throughout the body. There is no substitute here for experience, so try it and see how quickly you begin to feel back in tune with your body and, even better, re-energised.

Prepare by sitting comfortably on the floor. Try and keep the spine straight and, if you can sit in the lotus, half-lotus or cross-legged position, then do so. The important thing is to feel comfortable (sit on a chair if you like) so you can concentrate on the breathing instead of worrying, say, about that pain in your knee.

You must be careful how you seal off the right-hand nostril to start this breathing exercise. The yogis believe that different parts of the nostrils link subtly but directly with the chakras or energy centres in the body, and that clamping the nostril without regard for this can have an adverse effect.

Use the thumb and third finger of one hand to seal the nostril gently and remind yourself, before you start, there is no need for any force to be used. Now try it yourself.

To begin, gently seal the right-hand nostril with your thumb and breathe in through the left-hand nostril to a slow count of four. Hold the breath in the lungs while you switch to close the left-hand nostril with the third finger of your right hand, then release the air to a slow and controlled count of eight. Keep the left-hand nostril closed and breathe in through the right-hand side to a slow count of four. Hold the breath again as you switch nostrils and seal the right-hand side while you slowly release the air to a count of eight. If you cannot keep the breath controlled for a count of eight, cut back to four or six counts and build back up to eight. The breath control and quality are more important than the number you can count to.

To begin with, try and build up to 10 rounds of this breathing practice. You will feel the benefits immediately. As well as calming your mind and clearing blockages, both energetic and physical, this breathing exercise seems to reassure the body that everything is functioning as it should be.

Deep Breathing

In their excellent book *Breathe Free* (see Bibliography), the herbalist and nutritionist (respectively) Daniel Gagnon and Amadea Morningstar say that even the simplest forms of deep breathing help to ventilate the lungs and stimulate lymphatic drainage to speed up healing.

There are methods, particularly the Russian technique devised by Professor Konstantin Buteyko, which recommend the opposite. He argues that the root cause of some 200 conditions, especially asthma, is hyperventilation, where we take in too much air and breathe out too much carbon dioxide. It is true that some asthmatics who have embarked on the Buteyko programme have reported relief through shallow breathing exercises but as a non-sufferer and a keen student of yoga I am happier myself to practise techniques that have been tried and tested for thousands of years. Each day, whatever I am doing, I make a point of trying to remember to take three or four deep breaths every hour as recommended by Gagnon and Morningstar.

Dolphin Breathing

I used to swim every weekday morning before going on to my desk at the *Sunday Times* where I edited the Lifestyle health and fitness section of the popular Style magazine. Before too long, I twigged that whenever I was under particular stress, the nature of my swimming would change. I would forget about lengths or laps and find myself concentrating, instead, solely on the breath. It was as if I found a great release of tension by moving my swimming body in a rhythm with my breath. It might not look pretty to anyone dawdling about at the side of the pool, but what I found was that I gained even more relaxation, almost meditative benefits when I exaggerated this breathing pattern and spouted air, at the surface of the water, like a dolphin.

Imagine my surprise then when I stumbled across confirmation that there is no better way to release tension and relieve stress than breathing like a dolphin in water. In his book *Animal-Speak*, the animal expert and shamanic healer, Ted Andrews, confirms what I had discovered by accident, that breathing like a dolphin can bring great benefits. In a description of the power of dolphin medicine, he says the breath holds the key.

It can also, apparently, do wonders for your sex life.'Water is essential for life but so is breath,' Andrews reminds us. 'There are many different techniques for breathing and learning to breathe like a dolphin can not only help you become more passionate and sexual, it will also heal your body, mind and spirit.'

For the release of tension and stress, Andrews recommends you simply imitate the spouting breath the dolphin uses as it surfaces from the deep.

Keeping Lungs Healthy

Once you have improved the quality of your breathing, you can begin to investigate how diet and supplements can help keep strong lungs healthy. As well as vitamin C, another of the nutrients that is key to protecting all the membrane surfaces inside the body is vitamin A, which stimulates the immune system and which can be used in high doses – 30,000-100,000 international units (iu) – for no more than five days to beat a cold. For prevention, though, take just 10,000 iu a day.

An alkalizing nutrient which accelerates healing, vitamin A also has soothing properties that will ease an irritated throat. This is because it works to rebuild the mucosal lining of the lungs, promotes the lubrication of tissues and strengthens epithelial cells. Good food sources include carrots, dark leafy greens and sweet potatoes. In Ayurvedic medicine, pungent foods such as onions, garlic, leeks, ginger and chilli peppers are often used to help decongest the lungs.

How Minerals and Fish Oils Can Help

Minerals now being investigated by scientists who want to work out how nutrition can help prevent respiratory problems, especially asthma, include magnesium, selenium, sodium, copper, zinc and manganese. There is now a well-established link between a high sodium diet and an increase in asthma attacks. One of the jobs sodium does in the body is to help maintain nerve and muscle function. When there is a dietary sodium overload, the lungs of asthmatics have been shown to become supersensitive to the allergens that can trigger an attack. What researchers have also found is that a low sodium diet can improve healthy bronchial activity 1.5 times in men. (The same has not yet been shown with women, but then there are still only a small number of these studies.)

Magnesium is closely linked with sodium in the body. Raise the levels of one and the other will drop to compensate. In acute asthma, clinicians have found magnesium, which is destroyed by processing foods, has a dramatic effect; the scientific literature is now starting to catch up with this experiential evidence. For example, when a patient is admitted to casualty in the throes of an asthmatic attack, there is no difference in recovery rates when either magnesium or ventalin are given. In other words, this mineral can confer the same brochodilatory benefits as the normal prescription drug.

Blood serum levels of selenium, a powerful antioxidant which is believed to help protect the lungs, have been found to be low in asthmatics and, according to new research, taking paracetamol can decrease levels of another natural antioxidant called glutathione, which protects the lungs.

Researchers who compared aspirin and paracetamol in 664 asthmatics against its use in 910 people with no asthma found that those who took paracetamol every week were 80% more likely to have asthma than those who never touched it. They concluded that the paracetamol acts in some way to decrease levels of glutathione, resulting in less protection for the lungs. If you have any kind of breathing difficulties, then alcohol, which is a bronchcoconstrictor, will also be unhelpful.

A less well-known but highly promising mineral that can help keep lungs healthy is germanium, which not only helps deliver more oxygen to the body's tissues but actually works to generate oxygen production inside the cells. It boosts the immune system, which supports lung function, helps the body get rid of debilitating toxins and is now being used in cancer therapy, since if there is one thing cancer cells hate it is a rich supply of oxygen. They need an anaerobic, or oxygen-free, environment to multiply, which means germanium has the potential to starve a malignancy to death.

You can find germanium in garlic, chlorella and the immune-boosting Reishi and Maitake mushrooms, but if you decide to investigate a more reliable supplement source, practitioners say you must make sure you buy the purest form, which is called germanium bis-carboxyethyl sesquioxide-132 (thankfully shortened to Ge-132.) Cheaper versions may be tempting, but less pure forms have caused two fatalities and have been linked with kidney damage. As a result, germanium has been voluntarily withdrawn in the UK. You can, though, find it in cosmetics including face creams and bath oils (see Resources); it is also available in homoeopathic form.

The role of fish oils in keeping lung function good boils down to the fact that they inhibit the synthesis of leukotrienes, which the body needs to heal wounds and injuries but which, in excess, are believed to cause inflammations in conditions ranging from asthma to arthritis and lupus. Low levels of vitamin E have also been linked with high leukotriene production, so taking a good antioxidant that includes vitamins A,C, E and selenium, plus fish oils from an unpolluted source, should help keep the lungs in good working order.

Finally, if you suffer recurring respiratory infections, a supplement called Oralmat will help, especially if the transition between climates when travelling causes problems for you. It contains extract of rye grass, which is very effective for a range of breathing complaints, including sneezing, bronchitis and asthma. One patient, who knew her attacks were being triggered by environmental pollutants whenever she travelled by plane, described the remedy, which has been tested by researchers in Melbourne, as 'miraculous'.

As well as rye, which is said to clean and renew arteries and which is used in Traditional Chinese Medicine to reduce damp, watery conditions in the body,

Oralmat also contains energy-giving co-enzyme Q10, which is found in every cell in the body, and an immune-supporting substance called squalene which, in Oralmat, is taken from shark's liver but which is also present in olive oil.

Dirty Air

The air you breathe in contains about 21% oxygen and 0.04% carbon dioxide. The air you breathe out contains a fifth less oxygen and ten times more of the waste gas, carbon dioxide. If the air you breathe in is dirty, then the inside of your lungs will be dirty too. Pollution, which is now being blamed for the dramatic increase in asthma (in some regions, as many as one in four children now suffers), has also been linked to heart conditions and lung problems. And it is not just a problem of the traffic-clogged inner cities.

In the UK, for example, families who have deliberately left those smog-filled towns to find cleaner air for their young children to breathe were shocked recently to learn that even outside urban areas, air quality has dropped sharply. The environment charity Friends of the Earth has described the findings of increased pollution in rural areas as devastating – especially since, in Britain for example, some of the worst figures recorded and analysed were sadly taken from a popular nature reserve.

In your lifetime, your lungs will filter billions of litres of air. Tiny hairs in the nose are the first line of defence, but microparticles such as benzene and hydrocarbons can slip through, and any form of exercise in a polluted environment will exacerbate the problem. Cycle in the city, for instance, and much of the air you are breathing in (at the rate of 50 litres a minute if you are cycling fast) will actually bypass the nose filters and go straight to the lungs.

The lungs do have their own protective and cleaning mechanisms, but fine particles deep inside are difficult to flush out. Once lodged in the fibres of the lungs, these pollutants have been linked to cancer, bronchitis, emphysema, general breathing difficulties and a range of other health problems. Lung cancer is now the biggest cancer killer in the United Kingdom, and pollutants – mostly tobacco but including air pollutants – are to blame for an estimated 95% of all cases.

There is no real scientific evidence that trendy pollution masks will protect you unless you are exercising vigorously, and you may laugh at those who wear them to hoover the house or jog around the block, but if you are exercising in a polluted environment then anecdotal evidence from users suggests that they can help filter out some of the worst of these particles. (For suppliers of pollution masks, see the Resources chapter.)

Easy Air Pollutants Guide

Benzene/hydrocarbons: Hydrocarbons, including benzene, are emitted by car engines, but are also present in cigarette smoke. They have been linked with cancer.

Carbon monoxide: A potentially lethal gas produced by incomplete combustion, it disables oxygen-carrying red blood cells.

Lead: Effects build up over time and may hit the central nervous system. Some research suggests it can have an adverse effect on children's IQ.

Nitrogen oxides: Both nitric oxide and nitrogen dioxide are the products of fossil-fuel combustion. Sources range from cars and lorries to power stations. Both are constituents of that horrid inner city petrochemical smog and dissolve in water to make strong acids which corrode tissues. Effects include sore throats and runny noses.

Ozone: We may worry about the holes in the earth's atmosphere that leave us unprotected from the worst of the sun's harmful rays, but on the ground ozone itself counts as a pollutant which forms when nitric acid from nitrogen dioxide reacts with hydrocarbons. A reaction encouraged by sunlight, the effects range from a runny nose and sore throat to lung disease.

Sulphur dioxide: A nasty, acidic gas produced when coal or oil is burnt and which is part of the winter smog cocktail. Effects of high levels, particularly in asthmatics, include coughing and a feeling of chest tightening. Bronchitis, emphysema, lung inflammation and blood clotting have also been linked to this pollutant.

Suspended particles: Tiny solids found in diesel and coal smoke. The bigger bits get trapped by the body's defences, but tiny particles penetrate the lungs. Can be carcinogenic.

PCBs/dioxins: Generated by widespread incineration of solid waste. May be carcinogenic and may also have an effect on the central nervous system.

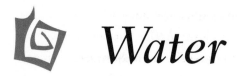# Water

You're not sick, You are thirsty. It is chronic water shortage that causes most of the disease in the body.

Dr F. Batmanghelidj, author of *Your Body's Many Cries for Water*

Dying for a Drink?

Dehydration is being hailed as one of the biggest causes of illness in men, women and children worldwide. You don't have to be stranded in the hot desert, parched with an agonising thirst and dragging yourself Lawrence-of-Arabia-style towards a shimmering mirage to be suffering this hidden health risk. You simply have to be one of the millions who fail to come even close to drinking the eight glasses of pure water that your body needs, each and every day, to replace the water it loses, to protect itself against disease and keep all your organs in optimum working order.

One clue to the importance of water to life is the fact that it is everywhere. Three-quarters of our planet is covered in water (all but 3% of the total volume is held in the oceans). This figure is then mirrored by your own body, which is also 75% water if you are an adult, and even higher, closer to 97%, for newborns. As a fully-developed human being, your 15 billion brain cells are mostly water (estimates range from 74.5-85%) and even your teeth are 10% moisture. You can survive for days without food, but just a 2% loss of the water surrounding your cells will result in a 20% drop in your energy levels.

A healthy cell absorbs nutrients from the water outside the cell, and the inner and outer water levels and contents are balanced by osmosis via the membrane of the cell. In simple terms, osmosis is the passage of a solvent (in this case, water) through a semi-permeable membrane which acts like a sieve between a less concentrated (weaker) solution to a more concentrated (stronger) one. Unless some outside force or pressure is exerted to alter the flow, osmosis continues until both solutions are the same strength.

In the body, then, the cell membranes are semi-permeable and allow water, salts, simple sugars such as glucose, and amino acids – but not whole proteins – through.

The Real Thing?

The pure genius of humble water as the key to good health first hit me when, several years ago, I chanced upon an article in a magazine called *Colors*, published by the Italian clothing company Benetton. In a special issue devoted to Fat, there were two photographs – one of a glass of water, the other of a darker liquid, a well-known brand of cola.

The headline was simple but carried a powerful message:

'You're thirsty, do you reach for the real thing?'

Which of these drinks, it asked, is the perfect nutrient to replace the eight glasses of water your body loses every day through sweating, urinating, defecating and exhaling? And which one contains the equivalent of eight cubes of sugar, makes you burp and rots your teeth? The caption explained how soft drinks are packed with so-called 'empty calories' – once you've burned up the sugar in them, there are no nutrients left – and how this trick sweetens the palate and sets up cravings in the body for high-fat, high-sugar junk foods.

About 16% of the total amount of water in your system right now is being stored in your muscles, which will become soft and flabby if you become dehydrated. When you realise that just the glands in your mouth, which work to keep it moist, use up to three pints of water per day, you can see how easily dehydration can happen.

The solution is simple enough – you need to increase the amount of fluids you are drinking. The trouble is, your preferred drinks – tea, coffee, cola drinks and even alcohol – are just not the right kinds of fluids. Alcohol, for example, is a natural diuretic. That means it forces water out of the body, causing the dehydration that is responsible for the worst hangovers (see Hangover Cures, page 162). In fact, for every alcoholic drink you take, you will lose the same volume of water from your body. Tea and coffee, too, are dehydrating.

Both the blood and the immune-supporting and cancer-fighting lymphatic system need pure, not contaminated, water to transport nutrients to cells and, just as importantly, to flush out toxins and waste.

So what should you be drinking?

According to natural health practitioners, the very best type of water for optimum health is distilled water. There are only three sources:

1 fresh organic vegetable and fruit juices.
2 water that has been distilled and purified by steam. You can buy the equipment to do this (see Resources for suppliers).
3 rain water that has passed through clean, unpolluted air.

Other practitioners will recommend that you install a water purification system.

Mineral versus Tap Water

You may already be drinking as much water as you can each day and you may have swapped your tea and coffee for herbal drinks and mineral water. Sadly, you may still not be drinking the right kind of water to keep your body healthy.

Over 800 chemicals have been found in drinking water supplies, including pesticides and antibiotics. There may be bacteria, nitrates – which will react with other chemicals to form potentially carcinogenic compounds in the digestive tract – and aluminium, high levels of which have been clearly linked with Alzheimer's Disease.

Simple, you say. I'll only drink bottled water. If only it were that simple! Some bottled waters pose more health hazards than some tap waters. Some are just tap water that has been filtered to remove the tell-tale taste of chlorine, and then given a fancy name. Even true spa waters may have been polluted. Tap water must pass 57 different tests for contaminants; mineral water can scrape by with just 15 assays. And, according to Anna Selby, author of H_2O – *Healing Water for Mind and Body*, European standards for factory-bottled water are actually lower than those set for tap water supplies. If you think this is bad, you will be even more alarmed to learn there are no tests at all for waters which are sold as 'Spring' or 'Table' brands.

Common contaminants include calcium, high levels of which are linked with a higher risk of kidney stones, and sodium, which most people now know can lead to increased blood pressure and a higher risk of cardiovascular disease.

In my house, we use a carbon water filter and a sophisticated water purifying system which works by combined reverse osmosis and de-ionisation to remove heavy metals, bacteria, nitrates and other chemicals from our drinking supply. With this system, our tap water is forced under high pressure through a semi-permeable membrane which prevents the passage of these contaminants into the tank from which we then draw a drinking water supply which meets the medical definition of pure water as containing less than 10 parts per million of total dissolved solids. Before I had this system installed, my supply was tested and shown to contain 400 parts per million of solids and other contaminants.

It often surprises guests when I drop to my knees and start filling their glasses from an extra tap hidden under the sink, but they invariably comment on the improved taste of the water they then get. It also means I am no longer drinking water from plastic bottles, which contain chemicals, including xeno-oestrogens, that are residual from the manufacturing process of the plastic itself and which have been shown to mimic oestrogen in the body and disrupt hormonal balances (see page 14).

Another common mistake is to think that eight glasses of a sparkling mineral water will bring you all the health benefits this chapter is promising. Sadly, there is a good biochemical reason to avoid carbonated waters: They contain carbon dioxide, which through a complex chemical pathway, actually works in the body to raise the pH of the stomach – making it less acidic and, therefore, less able to digest the protein foods you eat. This in turn can lead to malabsorption of the nutrients in your food.

The Big Fluoride Debate

Whenever I write about fluoride, my postbag doubles with irate letters from angry researchers and health authority administrators. I cannot understand why, when research has shown the same rate of decline in dental decay between fluoridated and non-fluoridated regions, we are even having this debate.

Fluoride is a cumulative poison, and while the body excretes about 50% of the fluoride we ingest, the rest is stored, mainly in the bones. Less than 2% of Europe's population now has fluoridated water, which was banned by Sweden and West Germany in 1971; Norway in 1975; Holland in 1976 and Denmark in 1977. France rejected fluoridation in 1980 – yet in the UK, over six million people still drink fluoridated water.

In the US, that figure rockets up to 135 million, despite the fact that groups as powerful as The American Cancer Society, the American Diabetes Association and The Society of Toxicology all stopped endorsing water fluoridation in the mid-1990s. These august bodies withdrew support following numerous large-scale studies reporting a link between fluoride intake and hip fractures, with some research showing an 87% increase among elderly populations. Skeletal fluorosis is now said to be a serious risk in people who have ingested 10–20mg of fluoride per day for between 10 and 20 years.

In the UK, an independent investigation of all the research into fluoridation by scientists at York University reviewed all the papers for and against fluoridation and concluded that the majority of those papers 'proving' it was beneficial did not meet the strict criteria of the peer review.

By the way, the US genius who first came up with the idea of dissolving sodium fluoride in drinking water in 1939 had no medical background and did not conduct any clinical trials to investigate the effect of this compound in the human body. Sodium fluoride waste, produced by the aluminium foundries at that time, was causing a problem on land and many of the country's biggest corporations were worried by the threat of expensive litigation and damage suits by disgruntled crop farmers and livestock producers. How they must have clapped and cheered when it was discovered that the children in a small Texas town where the water was naturally fluoridated appeared to suffer from fewer dental cavities. What better way to sell this toxic waste product as the new health hope?

You might know by now that tooth decay is the result of poor nutrition, bad oral hygiene and excessive consumption of sugary sweets and drinks, but as the US naturopath, Patricia Bragg, writes in her must-read book *Water – The Shocking Truth*, back then people were only too willing to believe that scientists had stumbled across a miracle cure to prevent all dental decay.

Ironically, some 60 years later, researchers at the University of Arizona caused a stir when they conducted a study which found that 'the more fluoride a child drinks, the more cavities appear in the teeth.'

Losing Weight

Drinking water before you eat will also help you lose weight. This is because the brain can generate energy from water and food. We eat to supply the brain with food and in response to a sensation that we are hungry, yet only 20% of that food ever reaches the brain. The rest, unless we exercise regularly, is stored as fat. When we use pure water instead of food, this storage does not happen. Excess water passes out of the body as urine and no weight is gained. The biochemistry behind the idea of water as an energy source may be complex, but try drinking pure water throughout the day (especially before meals) and watch the excess weight drop off. If you are not hungry, don't eat. Drink a glass of water instead.

Sacred Water

The Cherokee see and treat water as the earth's life blood. The Greeks revered water as the highest of all the elements, and in Traditional Chinese Medicine, where water is seen as the source of vital *chi* or energy, it is also said to link the five levels of human existence – physical, vital, emotional, mental and spiritual. Many indigenous cultures shared the belief that to look into running water was to gaze upon your soul and the face of God, and many authors have predicted that in this new century, water will become the most important cure-all in medicine and healing.

Most people feel physically and spiritually renewed and uplifted when given the opportunity to immerse themselves in water, and natural healers believe you can cleanse and re-energise your own domestic water supply, especially in preparation for bathing, by stirring the water in spirals as it flows from the tap.

In the 1960s, the Canadian researcher Bernard Grad experimented with water that had been treated by a healer and found it not only accelerated the growth of plant seeds but had an anti-depressant effect on patients suffering a negative outlook. Water also plays an increasingly important role in what many are calling the new medicine of the 21st century – Vibrational Healing – and in one of the oldest natural therapies, homeopathy. With techniques such as the Bach Flower Remedies and other flower essences, the energetic and healing essence of the plant is transferred, through the power of sunlight, to the medium of water.

Water has always played a role in spiritual rituals and meditation. When you meditate, sit facing North and place a small bowl of pure water to the West. This is an ancient Celtic shamanic and Native American healing tradition where the water signifies the emotions.

A Simple Cleansing Ritual

The Indian yogis, who live for years and who all look much younger than their biological age, use cleansing rituals to purify both the physical body and the mind. One of the more extreme is to use fasting and pure water only to purify the body and soul. One simple cleansing technique that you can easily incorporate into your everyday life, however busy you are, is called *Jala Netti*. It works fantastically well to relieve respiratory problems and prevent asthma attacks, and is very effective if you are prone to a build-up of mucus in the body, especially after eating dairy products. On an emotional level, it is said by the yogis to help you let go of deep-rooted anger and to release those energy blocks that may be holding you back in your life.

The first time I tried it, it made me cry – which I later learned is not unusual. It is also an excellent way to keep the nasal passages in tip-top condition, to resist infection and keep your immune system strong. Many people, once they get the hang of it, practise Jala Netti every day. Others only use it when they feel a blockage threatening or when, for example, they have spent the day in a polluted city centre.

Jala Netti – How to Do It

You will need a small Jala Netti pot. These are not expensive and can be bought from shops and suppliers which specialise in yoga accesories (see Resources). Find a screw-top glass jar (an old, sterilised jam jar will work) and carefully pour a tablespoon of natural salt into the bottom. Boil the kettle and, when cooled so that it is just warm to the touch, pour the water into this jar, over the salt. Watch the salt dissolve and stop, for a moment, to think about the amazing qualities of water as a solvent. (To liquify salt without water, you would need to heat it in a furnace to 800 degrees C.)

Now, pour this solution into your Jala Netti pot until the liquid comes close to the top. Take this, together with a pack of soft tissues, to the bathroom, where you are going to perform your Jala Netti cleansing over the sink. The idea is to cleanse both nasal passages by gently pouring the water into one nostril and allowing it to pass out through the other. To do this, you insert the spout of the Jala Netti pot into the nostril itself and tip your head to one side. If you are cleansing the right-hand nostril, tip the head to the left. Repeat on the other side.

Don't worry if it feels odd at first. You will soon get used to this sensation. Don't worry either if this ritual, which stimulates the *vagus* nerve that runs from the brainstem to the abdomen, with branches to almost all the major organs, makes you feel emotional. This is perfectly normal and is an excellent sign of the deep inner cleansing that is taking place and boosting your health and well-being.

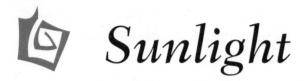 # *Sunlight*

The Greek sun god, Apollo was also the god of medicine.

The Big, Bad Sun

The sun has had such a bad press for so long now that we seem to have
forgotten sunlight was once highly prized for its many health benefits. Although
sunlight therapy was a popular treatment 100, even 50 years ago, a whole
generation of us have now grown up thinking we must keep out of the sun and
that we can only venture out safely if we've plastered our faces and bodies in
high-factor (and expensive!) sunblocks and creams.

Thanks to 20 years of successful campaigning by orthodox health professionals, a tan, for most people, is no longer perceived as being something healthy, no matter how good it makes them feel. And sunbathing, which we have come to believe is an almost certain prelude to cancer, is seen as being almost as irresponsible as smoking.

In the Western world, 90% of the population now spends 90% of their time indoors, which means the only time most of us ever truly get to escape what can seem like a twilight existence and feel the warmth of the bright sun's rays is when we strip off on holiday. Of course what happens the minute we hit the beach is that we forget all that sensible health educational advice, try and squeeze a year's worth of exposure into two short weeks and end up, not surprisingly, roasted red, raw and burnt, which really is a health hazard.

There is no question that unprotected and unaccustomed exposure to intense sunlight like this will burn most skin types. Scientists are convinced this can trigger one of the fastest-growing and frightening of the killer cancers, malignant melanoma, and we should not ignore the risks. But we have all been so busy worrying about the harmful effects of the sun that it has not occurred to most of us to stop and ask why sunlight (or heliotherapy) played such an important role in medicine before antibiotics were commonplace, or whether we could still benefit from it now?

Why, for instance, were young mothers in the 1960s so anxious to park those enormous *Mary Poppins*-type perambulators outdoors so their baby could get plenty of fresh air and natural sunlight, and why, we should be asking, was a scientific review of the medical literature – which concluded that 'the benefits of moderate exposure to sunlight outweighed by a considerable degree the risks of skin cancer, premature ageing and melanoma' – so effectively buried by all those anti-sun campaigns that few of us ever heard of it?[1]

Time for a Rethink?

The time has come to re-examine the facts. What researchers are beginning to rediscover is that safe sunbathing will *not* harm your health. Instead, it will positively provide a serious and sustained boost and protect you from a wide range of diseases including chronic skin problems and internal cancers.[1] If this is right, and sunlight really can protect against lung, bowel and breast cancers, heart disease, psoriasis and even the degenerative nerve condition multiple sclerosis (MS), then we all need to re-think our attitude to being out in the sun.

In his excellent book, *The Healing Sun – Sunlight and Health in the 21st Century*, the complementary health practitioner and sunlight researcher Richard Hobday, writes: 'Each year, lack of sunlight probably kills thousands more people than skin cancer.'

---

[1] IN 1992, DR GORDON AINSLEIGH PUBLISHED A PAPER CALLED 'BENEFICIAL EFFECTS OF SUN EXPOSURE ON CANCER MORTALITY' IN THE JOURNAL *PREVENTIVE MEDICINE*, IN WHICH HE REPORTED THAT HE HAD FOUND TRENDS IN EPIDEMIOLOGICAL STUDIES SUGGESTING THAT MODERATE SUNBATHING WOULD RESULT IN A 33% REDUCTION IN THE DEATH RATES FROM CANCER OF THE BREAST AND COLON IN THE US.

He knows this is a controversial claim, and one that flies in the face of 20 years of anti-sun campaigning, but he justifies his position by explaining something few people realise: Sunlight actually lowers cholesterol levels, and so is an excellent and natural tool for helping protect against heart disease.

Since this is still the No. 1 killer in the Western world, then even if sunlight has only a small protective effect, Hobday argues, the number of lives saved by controlled, safe and moderate exposure to the sun would greatly outweigh the number of deaths caused by malignant melanoma – but only, of course, once people know how to control their exposure and sunbathe safely.

The key word here – and the one that must be understood if you are to benefit in any way from changing your attitude to being out in the sun – is the word *MODERATE*. In other words, sunlight therapy only works when you go about it in a safe and controlled way. This means building up your exposure slowly and gradually. It does not mean booking a flight to the Bahamas after spending 49 weeks in a windowless office, throwing caution to the wind and allowing your poor body to sizzle.

Why Being in the Sun Makes You Feel So Good

The birds, the bees, my dog, my hens and even snakes do it, so it's hardly surprising that when the sun does come out, we all feel a pull to find a warm spot, lean back against a wall, close our eyes and worship it. Something happens when you turn your face or the back of your neck to the sun which simply makes you feel a whole lot better.

That something is no longer a mystery, thanks to our expanding knowledge of brain biochemistry. What happens is that sunlight triggers the increased production of the feel-good brain chemical serotonin, which, as well as controlling sleep patterns, body temperature and sex drive, lifts your mood and helps ward off depression.

The reason so many of us suffer from the winter blues or even a condition called Seasonal Affective Disorder (SAD) – which now affects 20% of the adult population – is that the body makes less serotonin in winter. Popular prescription antidepressants such as Prozac work to increase serotonin levels in the brain – and so does sunlight, which is why SAD sufferers eventually resort to an artificial indoor light-box treatment. What they should be doing, of course, is finding a way to spend a little time out in natural sunlight every day.

One intriguing new and as yet untested suggestion is that, during the summer, the body builds a kind of 'sunlight memory bank' to help those of us living further from the equator through the darker winter months. The theory is that the amount of serotonin your body produces in winter will be directly related to the amount of exposure to sunlight you enjoyed the previous summer.

Could it really be true that the amount of safe sunbathing you have done in the summer will determine whether you can keep the winter blues at bay once the days grow short and cold?

If you cannot wait for the science to tell you this is so, try a late sunshine break for yourself and see the difference it makes. One year, for example, I went to Antigua at the end of October. It was the first year I had been in a sunny climate so late on in the year and it was the first year I made it through a long UK winter and reached the end of February without thinking I couldn't bear another cold, grey and miserable day.

I know this is only anecdotal, but it was a promising enough result for me to pick up the phone to the travel agent when spring finally arrived to book a similar late autumn sunshine break for the following year. I felt, in some odd way, as if I had been more paced and even-tempered in my mood through the winter months instead of reaching March feeling depressed.

The Sunshine Vitamin that Is Really a Hormone

The pro-safe sunshine lobby – and it should be apparent by now that I count myself among them – have a powerful ally in the shape of a vitamin that is not a vitamin at all but a hormone: Vitamin D.

Sunlight triggers the body to make its own vitamin D, which is crucial not only for strong bones and healthy teeth but for keeping the immune system working.

Studies have shown, for example, that exposing the body to sunlight or even ultraviolet light from an artificial source increases the number of white blood cells, or lymphocytes. These are the body's primary defence against the onslaught of an infection, and are an important part of your immune response to the organisms that cause illness. Vitamin D also plays a role in increasing the amount of oxygen your blood can transport around the body – which, in turn, will boost your energy levels, sharpen your mental faculties and give you an improved feeling of well-being.

Few people realise the body also needs ultraviolet light to break down cholesterol, which may otherwise, at high levels, damage the lining of the arteries causing serious cardiovascular disease. Both cholesterol (which is needed to make the sex hormones) and vitamin D are derived from the same substance in the body: a chemical called squalene which is found in the skin. There is a new theory that in the presence of sunlight, squalene is converted to vitamin D, but without sunlight, it is converted instead to cholesterol.

Another reason sunlight is important to health is that you will only get a quarter of the vitamin D you need from the typical Western diet. The rest must come from exposure to the sun. You do not have to burn or tan to get the vitamin D you need. Just 20 minutes of safe sun exposure a day will do it. Of course, in some climates, there are times when this is impossible.

In the UK, for example, you cannot make vitamin D from sunlight between the months of October and March because the UVB radiation with the right wavelength that is needed to achieve this is only present at ground level from April to September. This means you are dependent on the vitamin D store you have built up the previous summer. This takes us back to the idea of building a sunshine bank and, if you live in colder climates, may prove your perfect excuse yet for a long holiday in the sun.

Without vitamin D the body cannot absorb calcium or use it for bone-building. Also, as you get older, your body finds it harder to absorb the vitamin D you do manage to get in your diet. While the recommended minimum dose under the age of 50 is 400 international units (iu) a day, over the age of 50 this rises to 600.

Lots of people think they can compensate for these problems by taking calcium supplements to keep bones strong or drinking a glass of milk each day. But you will waste your money on calcium pills if you don't get your 20 minutes in the sun or, if you cannot do this, take a vitamin D supplement to make sure the body can absorb it. Also, the amount of vitamin D in a glass of milk varies too widely to be sure of meeting, let alone exceeding, the recommended daily allowance (RDA).

Too much vitamin D can be toxic and predispose you towards kidney stones. If you know this is a risk, watch your intake of both vitamin D and calcium. Some prescription drugs, particularly anticonvulsant medicines, can deplete levels of vitamin D, so check with your doctor that you are not becoming deficient. Vitamin D is not toxic until you hit doses of around 2,400 iu per day – nobody needs or should be taking more than 1,000 iu a day.

The Skin Cancer Story and How to Protect Yourself

Here's a strange irony: Those countries which have taken the threat of skin cancer seriously and which have encouraged the population to use strong sun-protection creams over the last 20 years are reporting *increased* rates of malignant melanoma. These include the US, Canada, Australia and the Scandinavian countries. This rise is particularly marked in Queensland, Australia, where sunscreens were first introduced and heavily promoted by health groups.

There can only be one explanation – namely, that the prolonged exposure to sunlight that sunscreens allow, by protecting the skin from burning for longer, must in some way be triggering a greater cancer risk.

There are, of course, two types of burning rays, UVA and UVB. Both cause burning and tanning, but UVB was always thought to be the more damaging of the two, since it causes more rapid burning of the skin. In fact, until recently when it was discovered that UVA actually penetrates much deeper, health experts thought UVA was harmless.

What they now know is that not only does the UVA wavelength penetrate far more deeply, causing damage to the collagen that gives skin its elasticity, it is also more closely associated with malignant melanoma and premature ageing than UVB.

Scientists are now concerned that sunbathers may have been using high-protection creams which only blocked the UVB rays, and that this might explain why skin cancer rates have risen worldwide.

The simplest way to protect yourself from the sun's more damaging rays and to use sunlight to boost health is to learn how to sunbathe safely, how to build up your exposure slowly and when to stay in the shade and wear a hat when sunlight is at its most intense and likely to burn you.

Osteoporosis – The Silent Epidemic

If you need calcium for strong bones and you need vitamin D to make sure the calcium you eat can do its job effectively, then you don't have to make a huge intellectual leap to realise how important sunlight must be in keeping your very bones healthy and strong.

Vitamin D also maintains the balance between phosphorous and calcium and protects against bone loss by lowering excessive levels of parathyroid hormone, one of the chemical messengers which controls the breakdown of bone. Too little vitamin D and, as an adult, you are at risk of a condition called osteomalacia where calcium leaches from the bone matrix, leaving it soft. This can, if left unchecked, lead to osteoporosis – or brittle bone disease – which now affects one in every three women and one in 12 men.

Women naturally start to lose bone density after the age of 30. With men, this is usually delayed to the mid-50s. The menopause can accelerate this problem in women because levels of oestrogen, the female hormone which helps bones to absorb calcium, begin to decline. There may be no symptoms until a bone has fractured, and by the time you are at serious risk of osteoporosis, you may have already lost a third of your starting bone mass.

The World Health Organization (WHO) is predicting that the number of hip fractures, for example, could increase six-fold to over six million by the middle of this century. This is why osteoporosis is being described as an epidemic, yet one solution could be as simple and as free as safe sunbathing, because in studies of elderly populations who have suffered a broken hip, up to 40% have been shown to be lacking in vitamin D. There are also more hip fractures in winter, when bone density is at its lowest.

Other Ways Sunlight Can Protect You

In laboratory tests, vitamin D has been shown to slow down the growth rate of cancer cells. Does this mean that far from being the frightening cancer-trigger we all fear, sunlight could actually protect us from some of the cancers that are now responsible for more deaths in the West, after heart disease, than any other condition?

With a recent prediction by Macmillan nurses that cancer will affect up to one in two adults in the next generation, we need to find out why it is that death rates from many internal cancers increase the further you are from the equator. Why do malignant melanomas develop most often on body parts that are not usually exposed to sunlight – such as the back of the legs and the torso – and why are these rates higher in less sunny parts of Europe than in those closer to the equator?

In other words, why should living in warmer climes offer you greater protection from cancer – a disease that brings more fear than any other?

While epidemiological studies have shown, again and again, that this really is the case, nobody can explain why. The theory currently most favoured is that it would make good sense to investigate the link between sunlight and the stimulation of the body's own natural defence, the immune system.

How to Sunbathe Safely

So, how can you benefit from this wonderful and free health tonic? You know sunlight can heal and you know it can harm you. To enjoy the first and avoid the second, the single most important thing is to avoid burning at all costs.

Frequent, short exposure to sunlight is both safer and more beneficial than any prolonged exposure where, without creams, you will surely burn and where, even with them, you may be doing more internal damage than you think.

Early morning sunshine has been identified as the most beneficial, so get outdoors after breakfast. The full spectrum of sunlight is now recognised as being important to good health, so do not smother yourself in sunblocks and screens that filter out some of the allegedly more harmful rays. Instead, build your exposure up slowly and, if you are worried about burning, start with short exposures of just your feet and work your way up the body.

The recommended air temperature, when you sunbathe for health, should be below 18 degrees C (64 degrees F). Wear a hat so that the sensitive skin on your face, head and neck is safe, and avoid baking. You are not a cake!

The most important thing – and I will say it again – is to avoid trying to squeeze your sunbathing into the two short weeks of an annual holiday. Instead, plan ahead and pace yourself over the year, trying to spend a little time out of doors each and every day.

Remember, 20 minutes of safe sunbathing is enough to get all the health benefits we are now rediscovering.

ShapeShifting (Exercise)

When to Exercise

Researchers have now discovered there is a right and a wrong time to exercise. If, for example, you like to keep in shape by working out at the gym, then the best time to pump iron is between 5 and 7p.m. This is when your body temperature is highest, making the muscles and other body tissues more responsive and more flexible. It also fits with the notion of the internal bodyclock, or circadian rhythm. The bodyclock works closely with the brain cells and the hormone melatonin, which tells the body when it is time to wake or sleep. Exercise at any time of the day is better than no activity at all, but if you get to know your own bodyclock, you can maximise the benefits of the workouts you are planning.

First thing in the morning, for example, you will have more energy but your joints and muscles will be more stiff. Muscle temperature is low and exercise carries more risks. So, if you plan to exercise in the morning, make sure you warm up first and keep your routine light. Adrenaline levels surge around midday, which is a great time to work out if you can squeeze it into your schedule. This is the perfect time to do a high-energy workout and sweat off those fat-loving toxins. Avoid an intense workout very late at night, since this works against the natural bodyclock and can cause insomnia.

The goal of most exercisers – male and female – is a flat stomach. You may not want or even like a six-pack torso, but nobody likes a tubby tummy. Ask anyone who practises yoga or Pilates (pronounced pee-lah-tees) what they like best about these types of exercise and they will show you their flat stomach. They are proof that you do not have to crunch, grind or contort your body into painful positions but that you can build incredible abdominal strength by working with your muscles.

The reason Pilates works to flatten your stomach is that it exercises all the abdominal muscles at the deepest level. It also works on the corset-like *transversus abdominis* muscle to improve your posture, which then enhances your overall body shape. You could, for example, do abdominal crunches until you are blue in the face, but if your posture is rubbish, your stomach will still hang out.

I have no scales in my house because I think how you look depends mostly on how you feel about your current body shape. If you know you have been overindulging and feel heavy, then you do not need the needle on the scales to tell you it is time to take yourself in hand and burn off some of that excess fat.

Counting the calories is still one way to lose weight, but it carries with it lots of guilt (especially if you eat more than your allocation for that day or sneak in a chocolate treat) and anyway, it is not as healthy as changing to a more wholesome eating plan. It may be depressing but it is true that most people who lose weight by restricting their calorie intake put their lost weight – and more – back on. Those who stay trim by eating a healthier diet and adopting a modest exercise programme fare better at keeping the weight off in the long term.

Any exercise is better than none, but there is no need to punish yourself. Moderate exercise for say, 20 minutes, three times a week, will soon get you into a shape you – and your clothes – can feel happy with. Remember, the rest days in between are just as important as all those sessions in the gym, because it is when you rest that the muscles react to the stress of an exercise session and grow stronger to give you more shape and tone.

Walking

If the only time you ever stretch is to reach for the remote control from the other side of the couch, and if your idea of strenuous exercise is having to carry your own grocery shopping, then walking is where you need to start getting back into shape. It may seem uneventful but it can provide enormous health benefits, from strengthening the heart and lungs to building strong bones, hips and knees. It is easy and low-impact, which makes it safe – and it's free. If you walk with a friend, it will be sociable too.

A brisk walk can help lower cholesterol and the risk of heart disease. If you can walk about 10 miles (16 kilometres) a week and you walk fast enough to get your heart pumping, you can lower this risk by an estimated 50%. Fast walking can provide as many fitness benefits as swimming or cycling, but you will need to build up to this faster pace.

The only thing you need to get started is a pair of non-slip, shock-absorbing and ankle-supporting walking shoes. Start your new walking workouts by choosing easy and comfortable flat surfaces to walk on. On your first day, walk for just 10 minutes to get used to the idea of walking for its own sake. Build up over time to walking on gentle inclines, which will make the session more aerobic. Try to walk every day or at least three times a week. If the weather's bad, put on a raincoat or go walk in the mall. Walking each day will also help you to get the 20 minutes of natural daylight we all need to help the body make vitamin D, which is important for strong bones (see Sunlight, page 44). After six months of regular walking, you will feel stronger and be in much better shape.

Trail Running

Jogging may still be one of the most popular sports (in the UK it ranks No. 3 after rambling and fishing), but it is too hard on the knees for most people. Trail Running, where you run on soft ground over fields, through woods and pasturelands is a much better option. It is vastly more stimulating than running on the spot in a hot and sweaty gym, wondering how the model-type girl on the machine next to yours keeps her thong in just the right place, and for many runners it takes on a meditative quality and acts as a superb anti-stress activity. Better still, trail running burns 20% more calories than running on concrete.

So if you really want to completely change your body shape, then running is the best sport for you. I have, for example, seen 40-year-old women with the classic English pear-shape (heavy thighs and hips) streamline their entire figure within a few months, thanks to a regular 30-minute trail-running regimen.

To get started, you need comfortable running shoes that will support your ankles and a schedule which you promise yourself you are going to stick to. If you plan to be out running at different speeds and for a long time, you also need clothing (and plenty of layers) that will accommodate your body's changing temperatures.

If you have done little or no aerobic exercise for quite some time, do not make the mistake of limbering up and expecting to be able to jog around the block in one go. In fact, on your first venture out you are not going to run at all. Not one inch. What you are going to do is get used to the idea of being outside in your sports kit and familiarise yourself with the route you plan to take for your first-ever trail run.

On day two, you will run but only for one minute. You will cover the same route as the previous day, but will alternate running and walking. It is crucial to build your stamina and strength in this way, so be patient. One of the biggest rewards of running is how quickly your cardiovascular strength improves. Soon you will be comfortably running your entire route. Be warned, though: It takes much longer to build biomechanical strength.

The best thing about trail running for those of us who are exercise-shy is that it is anything but boring. You cannot get obsessed with your time, speed or performance because you will be too busy making sure you do not trip over a twig and too distracted by the fabulous views and the occasional glimpse of wildlife. If you feel you have become disconnected from nature, there is no better way to get back in shape and back in touch with the important things in life.

Swimming

This must be the world's most popular sport, so imagine my shock when, after 30 years of swimming, I got into a pool with an instructor who showed me how most of us have got it all wrong. Far from paddling up and down the pool, toning our muscles, releasing tension from our joints and exercising our pumping hearts, too many of us are unwittingly doing more harm than good.

After three lengths, one of each stroke (breaststroke, backstroke and front crawl), Julie Smith, a British swimming teacher and former Olympic backstroker, gave me the bad news: My breaststroke was a dated 1960s version, I was swimming the backstroke the way it was taught in the 1950s (I was not even born then), and my freestyle front crawl was prehistoric.

The good news, if your swimming, like mine, has become somewhat dated is that adults are quick to learn how to alter their strokes. With the front crawl, for example, the biggest change for anyone who learned to swim as a child in the 1960s is that overkicking is now frowned upon. The gentle kicks that are encouraged instead are both easier and energy-saving.

Learning the front crawl, I was taught to stretch forward with each arm as far as I could, brushing past the ear. Now you are taught to rotate the arm from the shoulder only, keeping the elbow bent and entering the water thumb-first.

The most significant change with the backstroke is that the shoulders now lift out of the water as they rotate to raise the arm, and the whole body rolls towards the opposite side with each armlift. This feels peculiar, but is not as ungainly as it might at first seem. Again, overkicking is out and the legs are used only for balance.

Of all the strokes, however, it is the breaststroke that has changed the most. Instead of keeping the arms close to the surface and reaching forward in a long, wide stretch, the hands scoop downwards and the shoulders and chest come out of the water. With this stroke, 60% of the power comes from the arms and 40% from the new whip leg kick, designed to get the most out of a powerful thrust of the legs. It is much narrower than the old-fashioned wide scissor kick that so many of us learned, and so feels completely different.

It may be annoying to discover your strokes are all wrong, but learning how to do them properly is rewarding because the newer versions are faster and more efficient. Only 2% of swimmers actually get any aerobic benefit from their swim – most do not even swim the 20 minutes that is required to get healthy because they become breathless – so it is worth learning the new strokes if they mean you can swim for longer.

The best new approach to swimming I have discovered is one that combines these powerful strokes with the Alexander Technique (see page 265), which teaches you how to improve your body awareness in the water.

Ironically, although it removes the emphasis on speed and getting to the end of each lane, this new technique increases efficiency in the water to such an extent that not only do your style and fitness improve, but so does your swimming time.

As well as highlighting the bad habits that slow you down in the water, applying the principles of the Alexander Technique also shows you the mistakes that can lead to serious longer-term health problems. The single biggest fault with all strokes is that of pulling the head back in the water and tensing up the muscles in the neck and shoulder. This triggers a chain reaction down through the whole body and can cause dizziness, headaches, strained chest muscles and even sciatica, where a nerve becomes trapped.

The impact of this gradual but persistent damage is actually worsened by the arms pulling against these tensed-up muscles. Pulling the head back causes the legs to sink, so not only is your swimming less efficient, you are also causing a kind of self-inflicted whiplash.

With the breaststroke, especially my 1960s version, the wide kicking of the legs can be detrimental to both the lower back and the cartilage around the knees, which, if the swimmer persists, can wear away, causing a condition known as 'breaststroke knee'.

The other problem that holds most swimmers back is breathing. Many swimmers hyperventilate, albeit unwittingly, by taking in too much air in a large gulp and then breathing out too little. The right way to breathe is to keep the face in the water, turn the head sideways and open the mouth to allow air in. Under the water, breathe out all the time. If you find this difficult, try humming aloud.

When we do get it right, water is, of course, the perfect weight-bearing medium for either getting back in shape or staying toned. The buoyancy, which reduces your body weight by 90%, protects you from injury, making this a great exercise option for anyone who has spent the last decade sitting on the couch or slumped over a keyboard. It is very soothing for stiff, arthritic joints and is the ideal form of exercise for pregnant women and anyone who is obese and who would otherwise be prone to injury.

Water aerobics are very popular and effective. More fun than exercising with your two feet on dry land, you will learn how to push against the weight of the water to walk on the spot and tone your legs and thighs, and how staying afloat and then exercising your arms and legs can burn off unwanted fat.

Swimming also charges the body's internal plumbing – the lymphatic drainage system – which has no pumps to drive it around but which relies on movement to flush out waste debris and toxins. It does not like aggressive forms of exercise but responds best to gentle, rhythmic movement. Stagnant lymph is at the root of many health problems, especially skin complaints, so if you want a good complexion, swimming is the sport for you.

Try not to develop just one stroke, because they all have different body toning benefits. The breaststroke, for example, tones the upper part of the body and the inner legs, but will exacerbate back problems. The crawl is a good aerobic exercise and will get the heart pumping, but if you are after serious levels of fitness you will need to practise the more demanding butterfly stroke. The backstroke releases stiff shoulder joints and is probably the gentlest way to get from one end of the pool to the other.

At the end of your swim, tone your bottom with a series of leg squats before you jump out of the pool. Hold on to the side, bend your knees and turn them outwards, and then drop down, rather like an inelegant ballet dancer. Hold the squat for as long as feels comfortable for you, and repeat until your legs grow tired. The body has its own innate wisdom and the more you trust this, the more you will benefit from your chosen form of exercise.

Yoga

I could write pages and pages on the shapeshifting benefits of yoga. If you are serious about toning up, sweating a little and finding your Moola Bhanda (the muscles which keep a tummy tucked in) then turn to Hands-On, page 255, and read about astanga yoga, which helped Madonna regain her fantastic figure after childbirth. Astanga, though, is not for everyone and even the less dynamic forms of yoga will help trim tummies, tone waists, lift bottoms and increase your overall flexibility. Having seen yoga being taught badly in various gyms and church halls up and down the land, I thought it was an exercise cop-out – but I was wrong. With the right teacher you are going to make friends with muscles you thought you had left somewhere in your more active teens.

Whichever type of yoga you favour, it will work on as deep a level as you choose. Force is never used, but you will learn how to control the breath to help tight muscles release, to stretch your body that little bit further and to master twists and leg raises which will help banish fat from around your waist. More importantly, what yoga will show you is that being happy with your shape is not about being fatter or thinner. It is about being strong, healthy and confident with the shape you are.

A lot of the postures (or *asanas*) take their names from animals to give you a clue as to what they are all about. The Cat, for example, is practised in Pilates too and gives the spine a wonderful stretch. It also works the abdominal muscles and lifts the bottom. The Cobra revitalises abdominal muscles which may have become lazy and stimulates both the liver and pancreas so your appetite improves. It also heats up the body to help get rid of toxins. The Camel tones the entire pelvic region and so is great for women, and the simple leg raises, which are perfect for beginners, strengthen the stomach muscles and break down surplus fat.

To get started, I recommend you find a good teacher in your area and take a few private classes. This means when you do join an established class you can really benefit from the postures and will not spend half the class worrying about the strange Sanskrit names of everyday positions which everyone else already knows. Yoga classes are excellent for overcoming inhibitions – nobody looks that good hanging upside down – and for helping you to feel comfortable with, and proud of, your body.

Tai Chi and the Magic Wand

Millions of Chinese men and women cannot be wrong. There is nothing more Zen-like than the site of a crowd of city dwellers, old and young, gathering under the spring blossom in a municipal park to practise their early morning Tai Chi exercises. A gentle, non-violent form of exercise that originated in Chinese martial arts and a Chinese philosophical system called Taoism, it consists of 108 complex and slow-motion movements that bring about mental, physical and spiritual harmony.

As with other disciplines, there are less well-known forms of Tai Chi. One of my favourites is the Chinese wand workout. It puts the emphasis on having fun as you learn to rebalance your mind and your body, so you end up feeling even more relaxed. The wand is a 4-foot bamboo cane, but if the budget cannot stretch to that, you can use an old broom handle. All the exercises you then perform are designed to make you healthier. As well as encouraging greater flexibility, they will lower blood pressure, promote good digestion and help drain the lymphatic system, which clears toxins from the body and which, as we have learned, responds best to gentle movements.

To improve digestion, for example, stand with the feet hip-width apart and hold the wand at the back of your neck. Bend forward slowly, releasing from the hips, as if moving into a bow. Keep the legs straight and avoid hunching the back. Hold this bow for a few seconds and move back into your starting position. (If you have done any yoga, a lot of these moves will come easily to you.)

All this bending and twisting with a stick in your hands is not as bonkers as it sounds. Canes or wands were used in Traditional Chinese Medicine as a diagnostic tool to pinpoint imbalances in the body, and can still be helpful in detecting underlying postural and muscular problems which, if left uncorrected, may lead to more trouble in the long term.

Whichever form of Tai Chi you decide to investigate, remember it is not demanding enough to give you an athletic level of fitness and will not increase cardiovascular performance, but it is the perfect shapeshifting exercise since it will make you feel – and look – taller, slimmer and more poised.

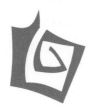

part two

Top-to-Toe:

An A–Z of 80 Ailments

and their Treatment

Introduction

When seeking natural and complementary health remedies, you are going to be investigating three main areas – nutrition, herbalism and homeopathy. Often, a holistic practitioner, especially a naturopath who treats illness without resorting to conventional drugs, will prescribe a combination of all three. It helps before you begin to take some of the reponsibility for your everyday health into your own hands, to know some of the basic tools and the reasons you are likely to benefit from the following remedies.

Nutrition – Why Take Supplements?

In a perfect world we would not need to take dietary supplements, but with food production and processing techniques that strip so many natural nutrients from the raw ingredients, we need to supplement our dietary intake to come even close to getting optimum levels of these important vitamins, minerals and trace elements. Self-diagnosing for everyday ailments can be helpful in the short term, but if the problem persists, and for more serious conditions, it is always best to seek advice from a qualified nutritionist or naturopath. A simple biochemical sweat test or hair analysis will reveal exactly which minerals and vitamins your body is lacking, a good practitioner will prescribe the exact amount you need to take. One big problem with the Do-It-Yourself approach is that these substances can work with and against each other, and so levels of one nutrient can affect levels of another in the body. This is what nutritionists call *synergy*. If you take a calcium supplement, for example, for protection against osteoporosis in later life, you also need to take magnesium.

I cannot understand why there is still any debate over whether supplementing a diet is helpful. My preference is to try the path of what I call 'True Nutrition' first, where you rely on natural foods to try and remedy the problem, but there can be no question there is an important place for supplements in holistic healthcare.

One of the counter-arguments is that there is no scientific research to support the growing use of vitamin and mineral tablets. This is not true. The research is out there but it is often fragmented, which means you just have to look harder for it. It is true there is not the same volume of research as for allopathic medicine. One reason for this is that companies which make and sell natural products cannot by law patent the active (natural) ingredient. This acts as a disincentive, since a small company could practically bankrupt itself funding clinical trials, but would then have no way of preventing other companies from jumping on the bandwagon and using that research material to make the same product but sell it cheaper, since it has incurred no research costs. This is an ongoing problem in complementary health, but with the recent explosion of interest in the field I am sure this will change and that, hopefully, companies will themselves adopt a more co-operative approach in the 21st century.

There is also no question that solid scientific research is effectively 'sat on' for years before reaching the public. Take the case of folic acid (vitamin B_9) and its proven role in preventing Spina Bifida and other neural tube defects in the foetus. The discovery that taking 400mcg of folic acid per day could reduce the incidence of this distressing condition by 80% is now cited as one of the greatest breakthroughs in 20th-century medicine. Yet, according to the authors of *The Natural Pharmacy* (one of my most well-thumbed health bibles), an astonishing 30 years passed between the time researchers first reported this breakthrough and doctors routinely passing the information on to their pregnant patients. The same is true of another discovery which could and should help reduce the risk of the Western world's number 1 killer – heart disease.

Homocysteine is a normal byproduct of the metabolism of protein, but high levels in the blood have been shown to be 40 times more accurate as an indicator of the risk of heart disease than cholesterol. When levels are elevated, it rapidly damages the arteries and causes an immediate build-up of artherosclerotic plaque – the main trigger for both heart attacks and stroke.

This link was first discovered by a Harvard scientist called Dr Kilmer McCully, who was investigating the cases of several infants and young children who had mysteriously died of advanced heart disease. His research, which won him no friends at the time, was first published 30 years ago. However, for political and probably financial reasons, his findings were ignored and McCully was forced to leave Harvard.

Perhaps the major sources of funding for heart disease research were only interested in those projects investigating the link between cholesterol and heart disease. This is bizarre, though, not least because 80% of all fatal heart attacks occur in men who do *not* have high cholesterol levels. A cynic might suggest the reason this information was suppressed was because commercially, there was less money to be made from a safe and natural supplement than from pharmaceuticals or cholesterol-free and cholesterol-lowering foods. The good news is that this injustice has recently been exposed in the US, where homocysteine research is finally getting the attention and funding it deserves. Sadly, we have yet to see the same trend in the UK.

You can, by the way, ask your doctor to test your homocysteine levels. If they are too high, you need to supplement your diet with vitamins B_6, B_{12} and folic acid.

Herbalism – How to Use Herbs

The fastest way to get the standardised, active ingredient of a herb into the bloodstream is by taking it in tincture form. This is always my preferred method when I am in a rush and don't have the time to grind, pulp or infuse fresh herbs.

You can also buy herbs and herbal combinations in tablet, capsule, powdered and dried form.

Organic Tincture Organic tinctures are now readily available in many health stores and by mail order (see Resources). Each herb will have instructions for how much to take and when on the label, so keep a supply in the cupboard for when you need them.

Infusion This is the method herbalists use when they need to extract water-soluble ingredients from the less dense parts of the plant such as the leaves, stems and flowers. You can also use it with the roots and fruits if these have been chopped finely enough.

What to Do: Pour 500ml of off-the-boil water on to 30g of the finely cut herb in a container with a tight-fitting lid. This coverage means that volatile substances which might otherwise evaporate are retained. Leave the solution for 10-15 minutes to infuse. Strain the liquid and allow to cool to body temperature. The usual dose is one cup of infused liquid taken three times a day, before meals.

Poultice This simply describes the technique where the fresh plant is bruised or crushed to a pulp which is then mixed with a moistening material, ready to apply directly to the area where it is needed. You can mix the dried herbs with a little hot water or use a host paste such as flour, bran or corn meal.

What to Do: To make a poultice paste, mix 60g of dried herb or herbs with 500ml of loose paste. Sandwich this paste between layers of sterile, thin cloth or gauze and apply to the wound or affected area.

Compress If you have ever placed a warm facecloth over tired eyes, then you have already used this technique.

What to Do: Soak a clean towel or sterile cloth in a hot or cold herbal infusion or decoction. Wring it out and place gently over the affected area. Repeat several times. If you are in a rush, you can use this same technique with water in which you have dissolved a few drops of your favourite essential oil.

Decoction The harder parts of plants, especially the bark, seeds, roots and rhizomes, only release their active ingredients after a more prolonged hot-water treatment.

What to Do: Soak 30g of your chosen herb in 500ml of cold water for 10 minutes. Pour this mixture into a saucepan, cover and bring to the boil. Lower the heat and simmer for 10–15 minutes. Remove from the heat, keep covered and allow the liquid to sit and cool for another 15 minutes. Strain and drink as a tea, in the same way as an infusion.

Homoeopathy

The principle underpinning homeopathy is that you use like to treat like. Thus, for the streaming eyes and running nose of hayfever, you take a remedy made up of the pollen of mixed grasses – the very cause of your misery. Technically, homoeopathy does not count as a natural remedy since the tiny homoeopathic pillules you will take have been synthetically manufactured, not harvested from nature, but the underlying principle of treating the whole person and the *cause* of an illness, not just the symptoms, brings the subject comfortably under the umbrella of complementary health.

In fact, homoeopathy can really come into its own as a truly complementary practice. For example, the first time I visited India, I decided to have the conventional anti-malarial treatments since I was a first-time visitor to this part of the world and because an earlier health problem had left my immune system under par. I was planning to travel in rural areas and did not think my immune system would withstand a malarial infection, so I took the allopathic pills but then supported my system with a tailor-made homoeopathic remedy to keep me well.

I rarely, in my columns, recommend more than the very basic homoeopathic remedies for more than the very elementary of illnesses. It can take up to seven years to qualify as a skilled homoeopath (as long as the training for many doctors) which is, to my mind, convincing evidence that this is not something you can pick up over a weekend course. A qualified homoeopath will, for example, take a detailed medical history at your first visit and prescribe according to what is known as your constitutional type.

Each homoeopath will have his or her own intuitive way of working, too. Mine, for instance, will decide on a treatment plan only after determining how the patient reacts to specific types of pain, as well as other factors. Hers is a very precise art, combining clinical training, experience and intuition. Your practitioner will decide on what is called a constitutional remedy. Mine is Gelsemium – and I am given this, along with other remedies, regardless of my specific complaint.

My feeling with homoeopathy is that if you can afford a qualified practitioner, then have a constitutional diagnosis and take advice for more serious conditions. For everyday problems, such as bruising or travel sickness, homeopathic pills and creams can be highly effective, so it is worth keeping these in your holistic medical kit as useful standbys.

In homoeopathy, the potency of the active ingredient of any remedy is so diluted that not only can it cause no harm, sceptics will argue that it can't possibly do any good either. New research is beginning to suggest the answer may lie in the fact that the human body itself is a natural homoeopathic machine.

Thanks to ongoing UK-based research, where homoeopaths have been investigating the ability of water to record a signal, it is now being suggested that homoeopathy works according to an even deeper principle than that of treating like with like. What is actually going on is something 21st-century healers call *Bio-Resonance*.

Bio-Resonance is a natural phenomenon and is what happens when, for example, you hit a tuning fork that has been pre-tuned to resonate at a particular frequency. It will only resonate at this frequency, regardless of how hard you hit it. What you will also notice is that anything else in the room which resonates naturally at the same frequency as the fork will also start vibrating. To the human ear, this will sound like a humming noise.

The idea, in health, is to think of normal resonance as being like a melody which illness or an infection shifts to a different key. When, for example, you have a sore throat you not only have the physical pain and symptoms, you are also conscious that you have a sore throat and, therefore, have become aware that you are ill. So, even with a seemingly trivial complaint, both the mind and the body are affected. What this means is that instead of just one particular resonance being out of kilter, the whole body has been disturbed. It then follows, if you accept this thinking, that if you are ill you will need a treatment (or, to follow the musical analogy, a series of tuning forks) which by resonating with your sick state will restore your original harmony.

Good health is maintained by this restored, natural vibration; when we lose it, through stress or shock, we are then vulnerable again to illness. Homoeopathy, it is suggested, mimics what actually happens in the body where vital organs, such as the beating heart, act as the tuning forks which impart that natural vibration or frequency to the body fluids. 'What we believe is that the signal or what we call the memory effect of resonance is recorded or held in the fluid of the body,' explains Tony Pinkus, the UK's leading homoeopathic pharmacist and director of Ainsworths, which is carrying out the new research. 'The implication is that the body is a natural homeopathic machine and this could very well be the long-awaited explanation of how homoeopathy actually works.'

Acne

Adult acne is not only a fact of life, it is on the increase. There are now 12 different types of acne affecting some 3% of the UK population. Contrary to popular belief, it is not caused by junk diets or poor hygiene but by a hormonal imbalance, the skin's reaction to this upset and a bacterium called *Propionibacterium acne*, which has become increasingly resistant to the antibiotics and other creams that are the conventional treatment route.

The dilemma for all acne sufferers is whether to go ahead and take the prescription drugs which, in many cases, can bring a dramatic improvement to the condition of their skin in the short term, or put up with the psychological trauma of bad skin while tackling the problem from the inside out. Roaccutane, for example, will indeed suppress your acne, but, for many, at a price.

You have probably read newspaper reports linking Roaccutance with depression and suicide in younger users. It works by shutting down oil production in the sebaceous glands, but its side-effects can include dry, cracked lips, nose bleeds, eye irritation, muscular aches and pains, hair loss, nail brittleness, high blood sugar levels and increased sensitivity of the skin to light. Roaccutane may also alter liver function and harm the unborn foetus if given to a pregnant woman.

If you are given antibiotics and you take them for a prolonged period of time, there is a risk you will, inadvertently, exacerbate the very condition you are taking them to treat. This is because antibiotics can also damage the lining of the gut. In one study, for example, tests showed 50% of those with a severe acne problem also had higher levels of toxins in their bloodstream. What this suggests is what the holistic skin specialists have been arguing for some time – that treating acne has to start from the inside. To replenish the microflora wiped out by the prolonged use of antibiotics, for example, take a probiotic supplement and eat bananas, which act as natural probiotics.

Teenage boys suffer spots and acne because of a surge in the male hormone, testosterone. In adults of both sexes, the same condition has been linked to the abnormally high levels of an enzyme called 5-alpha-reductase. Enzymes are the catalysts which trigger the body's chemical reactions. What this one does, unhelpfully, is convert testosterone to a more potent form called dihydrotestosterone, and it is this substance, which is now believed to play the key role in causing the condition.

As well as a hormonal imbalance, researchers have also identified an inability among sufferers to digest saturated fats. This means that eliminating dairy products and all animal fats, especially red meats, should help manage the symptoms. Both tofu and soya are phytoestrogens – substances which can help naturally rebalance the hormones in both sexes – and so eating these foods at least three times a week can help. Sufferers should also avoid yeast and white sugar. Women who develop acne-like outbreaks in their later 20s and 30s may also be suffering from a hidden condition called Polycystic Ovarian Syndrome (see page 203).

A calcium-rich diet has been found to help reduce the severity of an acne infection. While the obvious source is milk, if the lining of the gut is damaged, acne sufferers are likely to be intolerant to and unable to digest lactose (the sugar in milk), making green leafy vegetables, broccoli, tofu and shellfish better natural sources.

Vitamin A helps maintain all the surfaces of the body, inside and out. Good dietary sources include all yellow fruits and vegetables, unpolluted fish oils, and, of course, carrots. Zinc, which helps boost the immune system and which enhances the absorption of vitamin A, is lost in food processing or simply missing from non-organic food harvested from nutrient-stripped soil. Excessive sweating also depletes the body's zinc resources, causing the loss of up to 3mg a day. Foods that are rich in this mineral include shellfish, pecans, turkey and wheatgerm, so include plenty of these in your diet.

Foods for Acne

Eat calcium-rich green leafy vegetables and organic dairy products unless you are intolerant. Include broccoli, tofu and shellfish in your diet. Add rich sources of zinc, including wheat germ, peanuts, pecans, turkey and, if you're feeling flush, oysters. Eat bananas to help repopulate the gut with good bacteria that help flush out toxins. Avoid tea, coffee, alcohol and sugar.

Supplements for Acne

You should be drinking plenty of water – up to eight glasses a day – to flush out toxins. You will also benefit from taking B vitamins, MSM (organic sulphur, or Methyl Sulphonyl Methane), flax seed oil and zinc, all of which are known to nurture the skin.

Make-up that Will Not Make it Worse

The Canadian-born skin psychologist, Helen Sher, has helped thousands of sufferers worldwide with her skincare system which relies on water to rehydrate and soothe the skin. The Sher Skincare system is not cheap and will not work for everyone, but I've seen the before and after results with enough sufferers, young and old, to suggest you investigate it. (See Resources for full details).

Light Therapy

A UK-led study of some 10,000 sufferers is reporting excellent results using light therapy, with over 70% of those participating reporting significant improvement in their condition. The doctor pioneering this treatment, Dr Tony Chu, is based at the Hammersmith Hospital in London, England. He has dedicated his career to finding a drug-free and chemical-free treatment for acne. He has been widely quoted as saying his findings show light therapy is the most significant advance in the treatment of acne for two decades.

The treatment relies on the use of a device called the DermaLux – a kind of light box, which the user sits in front of for 15 minutes a day. The theory is that the bacteria which can cause acne can be killed by the right mix of blue and red light. Patients in the recent trials of this device also applied benzoyl peroxide cream, twice a day.

Allergy

Everything under the sun – including the sun – is a potential allergen. What is amazing is that we do not have more, not less, allergies.
Jonathan Brostoff, Professor of Allergy and Environmental Health,
University College London Medical School

It may have been around since 1966, but Enzyme Potentiated Desensitisation (EPD) remains a closely guarded secret outside allergy circles. Similar, in principle at least, to homeopathy, EPD works with the idea of treating like with like. Minute doses of allergens are given together with an enzyme called beta glucuronidase, which works in the body to increase and modify the effects of the allergen.

Beta glucuronidase is present in all parts of the human body, where it is released into the tissues during inflammation or an allergic response – in greater amounts than that given with EPD. With this technique, the dosage used is less than that contained in 1cc of blood from a healthy person, making it entirely safe.

There are two ways for EPD to be administered. With the cup method, a small area of the forearm is scarified to remove the waterproof layer of the skin, and the desensitising fluid is then held over this area, by means of a plastic cup, for 24 hours. The slow absorption of this dose makes this method extremely safe. Also, the immune system is much more responsive to doses through the skin than those given via injection. That said, the second EPD method is by injection. This is more reliable but may not be quite as safe.

Desensitising mixtures are now available for a wide range of allergens including pollens, dust, pets, moulds, candida, fumes, fragrances, foods and food additives. With EPD, many common allergens cross-desensitise in groups, which is good news for sufferers, many of whom are allergic to more allergens than they may have identified.

Over the last 30 years, EPD has been employed successfully to treat asthma, rhinitis, nasal polyps, eczema, urticaria, Irritable Bowel Syndrome, migraine, rheumatoid arthritis, petit mal epilepsy, chemical sensitivity, food allergies and intolerance, as well as the secondary allergies that complicate post-viral syndromes including Chronic Fatigue Syndrome and ME.

There is still no desensitising agent to treat allergies to insect bites or stings, contact dermatitis or drug-related allergies. Inoculating against the vast and ever-increasing number of chemicals used in the production of food has also proved difficult but common allergies, such as hayfever, can be treated with just one dose given about four months before the usual onset of symptoms.

Housedust mite allergy, the most common cause of eczema in adults, for example, can be treated with just two doses given over an interval of 2–3 months. It can take up to eight doses to establish a response, after which the frequency of treatment can be reduced. More than 50% of EPD patients have been able to stop any treatment at all for long periods – the longest recorded period without booster doses before a relapse was 21 years.

The response to EPD is four-fold. There may be an immediate response, or the full benefits may be slow to take. A reaction time of three weeks, during which there is either a 'cure' or the production of symptoms, is common. The main action usually starts after this, and lasts for 3–4 months. This is thanks to the immune system's allergen-fighting lymphocyte cells which have been created by the dose.

Some patients will have a very late response, from between 18 months and two-and-a-half years, starting from between 7 and 9 doses from the start of treatment.

A 'postpone action' has been recorded where between 6 and 15 months after the last treatment, the patient appears miraculously cured. Such patients have often given up on EPD, which does not work in any event for 20% of sufferers, and then attribute their miracle cure not to that last dose but to some other treatment.

EPD was developed by a British medical doctor, Dr Leonard McEwen, who has stuck to protocol. Follow-up studies and clinical trials all suggest this technique has much greater long-term success than any other method of immunotherapy. Word of its success has spread and there are now clinics and doctors in the US and Italy offering this simple but effective procedure which deserves greater recognition.

Altitude Sickness

If you are planning a high altitude trekking holiday, this may be your most serious health risk.

In its most dangerous form, altitude sickness is known as pulmonary oedema. This is the name for what happens when there is a build-up of fluid on the lungs and, make no mistake, it constitutes a serious medical emergency. The symptoms include shortness of breath and disorientation; those most at risk are smokers and anyone with an existing heart problem.

The secret to avoiding this problem is to acclimatise slowly, says the London-based naturopath and traveller, Max Tomlinson, who has travelled widely in South America and so speaks from experience. Do not rush your trek up the mountain, but enjoy this excuse to take your time and take in the glorious scenery, he suggests. If at any point you feel dizzy or short of breath, make your way back down to a lower altitude.

Tomlinson suggests that your holistic travel kit should include, as a precaution, two homoeopathic preparations, Aconite 6c and Arsenicum album 6c. Aconite 6c is used to treat the sudden onset of symptoms, including breathlessness, and Arsenicum album 6c should be taken if there is a delay between developing the first symptoms and getting medical treatment. You can take both at the same time and should take one dose, four times a day for up to a maximum of four doses.

Because there is less oxygen available at higher altitudes, you also need to make sure your iron levels are normal before you travel. Tomlinson recommends you take a liquid supplement called Floradix for a month, starting 14 days before you leave. Gingko biloba has been shown in clinical trials to boost the amount of oxygen and other nutrients reaching the brain, and thereis now good evidence that this too will help. Again, start 14 days before your departure date and take 20 drops of an organic tincture of the herb, three times a day.

There is also good anecdotal evidence for a homoeopathic remedy called Coca, which comes from the leaves of the cocaine plant. This will fall into place when you learn that those living in the region you plan to visit chew the same leaves for altitude sickness. The theory is that the active ingredient boosts the circulation of blood and oxygen to the brain.

Amalgam Fillings

More than a decade after scientists first began to question the sense of using mercury amalgam fillings, people with metal in their mouths are still not sure whether to leave their fillings in place or have them taken out. The simple answer is – unless you have an underlying sickness which may be linked with mercury poisoning – leave them in place until you need to have them replaced and then, whatever you do, don't let your dentist put such a toxic metal back in your mouth.

The silver fillings which have divided dentists for more than 15 years are not silver at all but are an amalgam made up of 52% mercury (older fillings contained as much as 75% mercury) with the remainder copper, tin, silver and zinc. Mercury, which the dentist must treat as toxic waste outside your mouth, is the second most toxic metal on the planet after plutonium and yet governments around the world – with the exception of Sweden and Austria – still deem it safe for fillings.

In Germany, amalgam fillings are only used for the molars, which are the back grinding teeth but in the UK, for example, the National Health Service will not pay for the more expensive white composite fillings, which means that although the figures for amalgam fillings have halved since 1986, British dentists are still putting 15 million metal fillings in the mouths of adults and children every year.

For a long time, the party line in both the UK and the US was that once the amalgam was in the mouth, the mercury became inert or locked in, and so was safe. Numerous researchers have shown this to be untrue, and practitioners do now accept that mercury vapour is indeed released into the body from these fillings. The current argument is that this seepage happens in such negligible amounts that the risk to your health is insignificant, although an estimated 3% of adults will be hypersensitive to this and will have an adverse reaction. Ironically, cleaning your teeth or chewing a 'whitening' gum actually makes the problem worse because it accelerates the rate at which vapour is released by a factor of five. Hot drinks increase the vapour concentration too.

Harley Street dentist and president of the International Academy of Oral Medicine and Toxicology, Dr Anthony Newbury, reckons he was the first UK-based dentist to introduce the idea of a mercury-free practice in 1979, after attending a lecture in the US where mercury seepage from fillings was linked, controversially, to chronic muscle and joint problems, fatigue and jaw complaints. He is a major presence on the international lecture circuit and says fellow dentists still accuse him of talking baloney.

'My response to the suggestion that the mercury vapour comes off in such small amounts that it is harmless is to say try changing it for cyanide, which is less toxic, and see how long you'll last. In science, even a nanogram is significant.'

Health problems which holistic practitioners believe may be linked with mercury toxicity include chronic fatigue, headaches, allergies and sinusitis, sore or bleeding gums, lack of concentration, memory lapses, irritability and depression – all conditions which could, of course, be linked with other causes.

It is also notoriously difficult to test mercury levels in the body because as it seeps from the fillings it oxidises into a form which then tightly binds with protein residues in the tissues, making levels difficult to gauge.

The Mercury Challenge test overcomes this problem through *chelation*. You swallow a chelating solution which will bind with the mercury before it can latch on to the protein. Your urine is sampled before drinking this solution and then again, three hours later, when it will be flushing out of your system.

I had my own mercury fillings taken out after reading that scientists at the University of Kentucky found the brains of those who had died from Alzheimer's Disease contained roughly twice as much mercury as the brains of those who had died at the same age from other conditions. They concluded these levels were far too high to have come solely from diet, and suggested that the mercury in their fillings was a more plausible explanation. Despite the fact I was paying for this, my then dentist grumbled his way through the procedure and, to my knowledge, did not follow the strict protocol which the British Society for Mercury-free dentistry recommends for the removal of amalgams, so be warned.

Holistic dentists say you can do more harm than good if you remove mercury fillings without proper protective procedures – which include using a rubber 'dam' to prevent the patient from swallowing any debris, including mercury, during the extraction, a nose piece with rubber hosing so the patient is breathing in air *away* from the mercury vapour that is being released, and damp gauze pads to protect the eyes.

A reported 95% of patients who do have their amalgam fillings out tell health practitioners they feel better. Of course, this is a self-selecting group, many of whom have suffered chronic complaints for years and who, sceptics will argue, are now blaming mercury toxicity as their latest fad.

I like the analogy one mercury-free dentist gave me: 'You could think of it like a battery effect sitting at the base of the brain, and when all the metal is out the brain is no longer bombarded by all those signals. It's a bit like switching the stereo off so you can hear yourself think clearly.'

Dentists and their assistants should also protect themselves – according to a report in the *British Journal of Industrial Medicine*, dentists have higher concentrations of mercury in the body and twice the number of brain tumours. Female dentists and assistants are three-and-a-half times more likely to suffer sterility, stillbirth and miscarriage.

If you do have your fillings removed you should also take nutritional advice, says Dr Jack Levenson, founder of the British Society for Mercury-free Dentistry. Charcoal tablets, for example, will help 'mop up' any mercury that does find its way into your stomach. If you plan to have your amalgam fillings out, start taking 2–5g of charcoal tablets for two days before the procedure and for a week afterwards. You also need extra vitamin C to boost your immune system, and selenium (a potent antioxidant) which works to detoxify mercury.

The Canadian researchers who first began to investigate the health hazards of mercury in the mouth started their trials by looking at what happened to the mercury from fillings in the mouths of sheep. They found that, within 30 days, mercury had accumulated to such an extent in the kidneys that their function was reduced by 50%. (The same test using a white plastic filling had no effect on kidney function.)

Critics ridiculed these studies, pointing out that sheep have different chewing patterns from humans. The Canadian researchers did the same experiments with monkeys and found, again, that mercury did accumulate in the body, but this time in higher doses in the jaw, the colon and the large intestine. The monkeys also had smaller (but still enormous) amounts of mercury in their kidneys than the sheep.

Dental amalgams remain the most controversial of all dental issues, but a growing number of practitioners admit they find it increasingly hard to argue with the opening statement of a book called *The Mercury in Your Mouth* which claims: 'Chronic mercury toxicity from "silver" mercury amalgam dental fillings is the most important, unrecognised health problem of our time.'

Antibiotics – Alternatives: Colloidal Silver

While most antibiotics disinfect only about half a dozen germs, silver has been reported to disinfect well over 600 different strains. Even better, infections which can become resistant to antiobiotics cannot develop the same defence against silver, making it an excellent alternative to antibiotics.

A *colloid* is a substance that consists of ultra-fine particles suspended in a different medium; in the case of colloidal silver, this medium is water. The particles are so small – 0.001 to 0.0001 of a micron in diameter – that colloidal silver is completely safe to use both internally and externally. I was first prescribed it for a persistent candida infection after a long hospitalisation, and there is no question that it worked.

Before the advent of antibiotics, colloidal silver was given in just about every way modern drugs are administered, but it fell out of fashion when practitioners started to prescribe hundreds of times the correct dosage – which led, in some cases, to a grey skin discolouration. Slowly, it has been finding its way back, and although nobody knows exactly how it works, the most accepted theory is that it targets and then disables the enzymes which many forms of bacteria, fungi and viruses need for their own metabolism and survival.

In recent laboratory tests, scientists found that colloidal silver was effective against many of the more insidious organisms including *Staphylococcus aureus*, *Salmonella typhi* and *Candida globata*. Jane Waters, holistic skin specialist, co-founder of The Alternative Centre (see Resources) and a researcher into complementary health, points out that in India, where people understand that silver acts as a natural antibiotic, it is still traditional to keep water in silver jugs.

Colloidal silver, she says, is excellent for treating skin problems such as athlete's foot, ringworm, impetigo and boils, but the purity of the product you use is important. Find one that has no binding agents, stabilisers or added proteins.

If you're not sure, ask before you buy. A quality manufacturer will have nothing to hide, and a good retailer should be able to source the purest colloidal silver available.

Arthritis

Almost half the population over the age of 65 will suffer some form of arthritis – an umbrella term for some 200 different debilitating joint and muscular problems. The two most common forms are rheumatoid arthritis and osteoarthritis. Both are on the increase, and both are increasingly recognised as the result of chemical lifestyles coupled with poor nutritional choices.

Since the 1940s, for example, the use of chemicals in the production of food has increased 10-fold, yet only about 1% of the produce in the supermarkets will have been tested for contaminants, including pesticide residue. When such chemicals do get into the body, they break down or combine with other molecules to form damaging metabolites. These, and other waste products, are carried in the bloodstream but dumped in the muscles and joints where they can crystallise, causing inflammation and the symptoms of rheumatoid arthritis. (See Dietary Cleansing on page 135 for a nutritional solution that works. It is strict but it gets results.)

Osteoarthritis is caused by the wear and tear of connective tissue, particularly cartilage, around the joints. This tissue normally retains water to act as a shock absorber, but once damaged it can no longer do this and instead, leaves the bones exposed, resulting in pain, stiffness and swellings. Early signs of arthritis include muscular aches and pains, stiffness in the joints and swelling.

There is no single cure for any of the different types of arthritis. What works for one person may do nothing for another but avoiding chemicals in your food by switching to an organic diet can help, as will managing the symptoms with a programme of moderate exercise, anti-inflammatory herbs and foods and collagen-building supplements. Lots of people take fish oils (which provide omega-3 fatty acids) to help alleviate stiffness. If you take this option, make sure your fish oils come from an unpolluted source. If you are not sure, check with your health practitioner.

Glucosamine is the substance many sufferers now swear by, but while it can bring relief it does not work for everyone. It takes several months to kick in, (which makes prescription anti-inflammatory drugs a more appealing rapid solution to the pain) and is still a long way from being that miracle cure. It is a natural constituent of cartilage and has been shown to stimulate the production of connective tissue, prompting claims that it will not only halt the progress of the disease but also reverse it by re-building lost cartilage. Sadly, the body's own levels of glucosamine decrease with age.

What has now been proven is that glucosamine works best when taken in conjunction with chondroitin, a substance which attracts more fluid into the spaces around the joints to lubricate them. Early results of trials in Germany show it is also very effective when taken with collagen, an essential protein which is crucial for building bone. There are now new supplements on the market which combine all three active ingredients.

Daily doses of vitamin D (400iu) and high doses of vitamin E (2500iu) have also been shown in various studies to slow down the disease and reduce the symptoms of arthritis. (Do not take high doses of vitamin E if you have heart problems.) So have daily doses of borage oil, which contains a joint-protecting substance called Gamma Linolenic Acid (GLA). One trial showed that those taking the equivalent of 2.4g daily, alongside their regular arthritis drugs, were six times more likely to report a significant improvement in joint pain and swelling than those in a control group. In the second six months of the year-long study, 50% of those taking high doses of GLA reported a 50% reduction in pain and stiffness. Unfortunately, borage oil also contains uresic acid, so long-term use is ill-advised.

Another fatty acid, found in small quantities in foods such as nuts, vegetables and butter, is Cetyl Myristoleate (CM). There are no double-blind clinical trials investigating its usefulness in the treatment of arthritis, but researchers are excited by the discovery that Swiss albino mice, which are born with unusually high levels of this fatty acid, never get arthritis and seem to be protected even when exposed to factors which cause the condition in other breeds. Of course, what works for mice may not work for men.

Organic sulphur, or Methyl Sulphonyl Methane (MSM), is also crucial to healthy connective tissue. It is found in every cell in the body and plays a key role in the production of amino acids, which are the building blocks of protein. Although available in a wide range of foods, including plants, meat, eggs, poultry and dairy, it can be destroyed by heat and food processing – so to relieve the pain and inflammation of arthritis, try taking it in supplement form.

Digestive health plays a role in relieving the symptoms of arthritis, too. Researchers admit they have no idea why this should be the case, but a deficiency of the so-called 'friendly' bacteria, which aid digestion in the gut has now been linked with a worsening of symptoms. To remedy this, you need to take a good probiotic supplement such as *Lactobacillus acidophilus*.

Foods that Can Help

An Indian take-away is not an obvious health food, but a curry can actually help alleviate joint problems. This is because its spices, which usually include turmeric, cardamom, cinnamon, garlic, ginger, coriander and cumin, all have an anti-inflammatory action in the body.

Chillies are another fiery food, which can help. They contain a chemical called capsaicin, which lowers levels of another chemical called substance P, normally used to send pain signals around the body. Capsaicin also triggers the release of the body's own pain-relieving endorphins, which work in the same way as morphine.

Anchovies contain omega-3 fatty acids, which also modulate the metabolism of prostaglandin. Too much of the latter, which plays a part in inflammatory conditions, can make the symptoms worse. Foods that may exacerbate your symptoms and which should, therefore, be reduced, include the nightshade family. This means cutting down on tomatoes, potatoes and aubergines.

Asthma

There are lots of excellent books devoted solely to this subject, but with an alarming increase the number of adult asthma cases and with growing evidence that asthma drugs themselves can exacerbate the problem by interfering with normal lung functioning (making them more sensitive to the allergens that trigger an attack), it more than merits a mention. Also, read Allergy (page 84), which describes a technique called Enzyme Potentiate Desensitisation (EPD) that has achieved excellent results with all allergy-induced conditions, including asthma.

To identify the allergens that trigger your asthma, you need to examine emotional, environmental and hereditary factors. The most common one, of course, is housedust and the housedust mites that live in furniture and bedding. Mould spores and animal detritus are a problem, or it may be DIY chemicals and other household or workplace irritants that are to blame.

You may also need to re-examine what is on your dinner plate. Many studies now indicate that food allergies are just as likely as environmental pollutants to trigger asthma in children and in adults. When researchers compared asthma rates among children living on the unpolluted Scottish Isle of Skye, for example, with those living in the Scottish town of Aberdeen, they found the incidence rate on the relatively unpolluted island much higher (17%) than in Aberdeen or when compared to the national average (11%).

Anaphylaxis is the extreme allergic and sometimes fatal reaction to an allergen. New figures show that this type of reaction triggered by food is on the increase, and that a big part of this reaction is usually an asthmatic attack. In Barcelona, for instance, doctors were astonished to find certains days of the week becoming asthma 'epidemic' days. The hospitals would be crowded out with sufferers, who had both a rapid onset of symptoms and a rapid recovery rate. It was then discovered that these epidemic days coincided with the offloading of soya-bean products at the docks. The solution was simple: Special filters were attached to the dockside silos and the asthma epidemic days ended.

In another clinical study of asthmatic children, those given 1,000mg of vitamin C each day for two weeks had less than a quarter as many asthmatic attacks as those given a placebo. For adults, the recommended dosage is increased to 2g a day and raised to 4–7g during a reaction. (At this high dosage, diarrhoea is a likely side-effect.) Vitamin B_{12}, particularly via intramuscular shots, has been shown to reduce asthmatic symptoms dramatically. In one study of 85 patients, all sufferers benefited from a 1,000mcg dose of B_{12} at weekly intervals. The younger the patient, the better the response, with 83% of children under the age of 10 showing marked improvement.

The figures for childhood asthma have doubled in recent years (in some regions, as many as one in four children will now be asthmatic), and while we now know much more about the mechanism of asthma, nobody seems any closer to a cure. Homeopathic immunotherapy has produced excellent clinical results in the treatment of asthma in children. In a French study of 182 children aged between 2 and 8, for example, the homoeopathic remedy *Poumon histamine* was shown to reduce the number of severe asthma attacks. This would always be my starting point in tackling the problem of asthma in young children, since children (and animals) respond exceptionally well to homoeopathy, which is also completely safe.

Bad Breath

If your dentist cannot find an explanation for persistent bad breath, then you need to turn your attention to your diet and digestive process. Pockets of infection in the gums are an obvious dental cause of halitosis, but many holistic practitioners will also investigate the possibility of abnormal fermentation of food in the gut. This will be exacerbated by dairy products, so cut these out of your diet for a week and see if your breath improves.

You may also need to take an anti-Candida (Thrush) approach to eating, which means eliminating all refined carbohydrates, sugars and yeast-based products too. If you have taken antibiotics in the past, these may have disturbed the balance of the so-called good bacteria in the gut, which aid the digestive process and prevent the fermentation of undigested food particles. To rebuild these, take a good quality probiotic (see page 171), which will contain millions of replacement live bacteria, plus a supplement called Fructo-oligosaccharide (FOS), which will provide food for these organisms and help cleanse the bowel.

A digestive enzyme may also prove beneficial – take one at the end of each meal. The friendly bacteria in the digestive tract flourish in a more alkaline environment. Help create this by taking one eighth of a teaspoon of pure sodium bicarbonate 20 minutes after eating.

The high chlorophyll content of parsley makes it a natural breath freshener. In ancient Rome, people would chew parsley to disguise the smell of alcohol on their breath. Chlorophyll converts carbon dioxide to oxygen in the body and helps lubricate the digestive tract, especially the various valves which, when working optimally, prevent gases and toxins from backing up the tract. The Greeks preferred to chew on Anise seeds, which taste of liquorice. You may prefer the taste of fennel seeds. A simple decoction (see page 76) made up of 2 lavender flowers, 2 sage leaves and myrrh resin will also alleviate symptoms. Gargle with this mixture three times a day. Aloe Vera is also an excellent colon cleanser and will help prevent an accumulation of toxins. Buy a brand that is high in mucopolysaccharides, the active ingredient. If the label does not give you this information, ask your healthfood retailer or contact the manufacturer direct.

Bloating

The bitter-tasting herb, gentian, not only aids digestion by stimulating increased salivary flow and gastric juices, but also reduces bloating. It is one of the best stomach tonics in natural medicine and also helps strengthen the pancreas and the spleen. Either take it as an organic tincture or make your own fast-acting herbal tea by brewing half a teaspoon of powdered gentian root with half a cup (125ml) of boiling water for 5 minutes. Strain the mixture and drink 30 minutes before eating. If the taste is too unpalatable, sweeten with a little honey or organic maple syrup.

Where bloating is linked with pre-menstrual tension, the Chinese herb dong quai, together with black cohosh, liquorice, ginger and uva ursi, can all help ease the discomfort. Animal studies have shown that ginger, for example, increases the gut's peristaltic action to aid elimination. Liquorice, which has been used medicinally since Roman times, acts as a mild laxative but has antispasmodic properties too. For a tailor-made, safe herbal remedy combining all these, consult a qualified herbalist (see Resources). Avoid liquorice if you suffer from hypertension, arrhythmias and any renal or liver disease.

Many practitioners believe that hidden food allergies or intolerances are now responsible for undiagnosed symptoms, including bloating, and that this problem may be affecting up to 60% of all adults. The main cause appears to be the regular consumption of a limited number of foods, coupled with impaired digestion and elimination. One of the biggest offenders is wheat, so if you do tend to bloat, and no other underlying medical cause has been identified, it makes sense to take steps to cut this food from your diet.

You are more likely to have a cyclical rather than a fixed allergy. This means that after avoiding a particular food (such as wheat) for a period of time (usually for around four months), you can then slowly re-introduce it as long as you limit the amount you eat. If your allergy is fixed, nothing you do will make you more tolerant of the allergen, so once you have identified it, cut it out for good. (See page 84 for more on allergies.)

The simplest way to check for food intolerance is to adopt an elimination diet for between one week and one month. This would include, typically, lamb and chicken (if you eat meat), potatoes, rice, bananas, apples, cabbage, brussels sprouts, broccoli and other members of the cabbage family. If your bloating is food-related, the symptoms should disappear by the sixth or seventh day of this diet and will reappear when you reintroduce the offending foods. Keep a food diary to help identify all the foods you may be hypersensitive to. Try this elimination programme with wheat, for example, and watch your stomach miraculously flatten within the week!

Blushing

If you suffer from embarrassing blushing, you are the perfect candidate for a homeopathic remedy. A qualified homoeopath can make what is called a constitutional diagnosis based on your physical and psychological make-up before prescribing the right remedy, but if you want to self-prescribe, take a remedy called Pulsatilla which is also known as windflower (the flower is often too heavy for the stalk and so gets blown about by the wind, hence the nickname) or anemone.

Patients who respond well to this remedy tend to be shy and clingy. They crave sympathy and often feel tearful too. The flower of this plant is also highly coloured, which herbalists and homoeopaths interpret as another 'signal' that it is suited to helping someone who is prone to blushing. You may also benefit from homoeopathic Phosphorous, which is often prescribed to people who are lively and outgoing but who may have a tendency to hypochondria. These types also blush easily.

Boils

If you suffer recurrent boil infections, you need to take a long look at your lifestyle. Poor nutrition and an overload of stress will depress the immune system, making you more susceptible to an infection by the *Staphylococcus* organism that is usually responsible for this skin problem.

Several potent herbs will act not only as blood cleansers, but as antibacterial agents to help prevent re-infection too. Cutting out stimulants such as tea, coffee, alcohol, sugar, sweets and cakes will greatly relieve some of the burden on your immune system. If you cannot give them up, try and cut down on these if you can.

If you have an infection, bring the boil gently to a head using either pure tea tree oil, applied two or three times a day, or by making a hot poultice mixing calendula tea and slippery elm powder. (To make a poultice, mix the herbs with boiling water to form a paste. Spread the paste on clean cloth and, when it is no longer scalding, apply to the boil. Cover with a thick towel to keep the site hot.)

The concentration of the active ingredients in commercial tea tree products varies wildly. To treat a boil, find the purest product you can. A native of coastal Australia where the traditional aborigine healers used tea tree to treat cuts, burns and athlete's foot (see page 93) tea tree oil is five times stronger than any household disinfectant and yet entirely safe to use on skin. Although it contains some 48 different compounds, the main active ingredient is called terpinen-4-ol. It has both antibacterial and antifungal properties and, according to current tests, may even prove effective against *Staphylococcus aureus*, one of the antibiotic-resistant so-called Superbugs. Tea tree oil, which is distilled from the leaves of the plant, can actually dissolve pus and debris lodged in the skin, but it can also cause drowsiness if ingested and should be avoided if you are pregnant or breastfeeding.

You may only think of alfalfa as a veggie-style sandwich filling, but with roots that can penetrate more than 60 feet down into the earth it is one of nature's own superfoods and very effective in treating skin problems. Alfalfa contains all the vitamins and minerals known to man, it helps build blood and is high in vitamin A, which is crucial for healthy skin and maintaining the body's mucus membranes. Black walnut, a traditional treatment for syphilis, is rich in both organic iodine and silicon, which will also help keep skin healthy.

I am prone to skin problems, especially when feeling stressed or run down, and I always supplement my diet with bioflavanoids. Taken with vitamin C (500mg a day) and zinc (15mg), these promote wound healing and reduce scarring. Bioflavanoids give fruits and vegetables their colouring. There are more than 500 of them, many of which are now believed to have excellent disease-fighting properties.

A good antioxidant to provide extra vitamins A, C and E plus selenium will also help, as will a diet that is rich in fresh fruits and vegetables, especially dark, leafy greens. As a fan of juicing (see page 8), which will get large numbers of nutrients into the system in a small volume of liquid, I recommend you try carrot, cabbage, celery, apple, parsley, blueberries, bilberries, any of the other dark, shiny berries and any of the citrus fruits. These will all bolster your body's defences. Members of the sulphur-rich cabbage family are important, too. Sulphur has natural antibacterial properties and can help keep skin clear. You can also take organic sulphur (Methyl Sulphonyl Methane) in supplement form. If you do, watch your hair, skin and nails improve!

Invest in a soft body brush to use for dry skin brushing after a bath or shower. Work the brush in upward, circular motions on the skin to stimulate the lymph system and prevent it from dumping a toxic overload on the skin. If you really want to kick-start your lymphatic drainage, take a deep breath and alternate hot and cold showers with skin brushing.

For a herbal remedy to prevent or treat boils, consult a qualified herbalist. I also found acupuncture very helpful, and although I usually recommend a constitutional diagnosis by a qualified homoeopath, there are DIY-remedies which will help reduce the pain and swelling when you have an infection. In the early stages, for example, Belladonna 30c will help. If you want to bring the boil to a head, try Hepar sulp. 6c.

Recurrent infections can also be a sign of diabetes, so check with your doctor.

Cancer

There are so many excellent books explaining how complementary health can help protect against and even treat cancer that it would be an insult even to attempt to broach the subject here. What I do want to do, though, is mention two of the so-called 'fringe' treatments that I believe all cancer patients should at least know about if they are to make truly informed treatment choices. You may have cancer or know someone who has, but the chances are you will not have heard of either of these treatment programmes.

The first is called The Gerson Therapy, after Dr Max Gerson, a German army surgeon who was working in the 1950s and who first experimented with nutrition and health in an attempt to control his own migraine attacks.

Through trial and error, Gerson hit upon a fresh fruit and raw vegetable diet that was high in potassium and low in sodium. It stopped his headaches, and so he began to prescribe it to patients who suffered the same problem. He then discovered, quite by chance, that the diet also cured TB in a patient who happened to suffer from both conditions, but it did not occur to him to suggest it for cancer until a female patient with the disease insisted he let her try it. Gerson knew this was a long shot but, to his surprise, it worked and the patient lived.

He could not explain to his colleagues how a diet could cure both cancer and TB, but what he could show was that his results were always much better in cases where there had been no prior orthodox treatment. He started to treat many cancer patients, explaining his theory that when the metabolism is healthy, cancer cells cannot survive.

The key to this innate health is the liver, and so the Gerson Therapy detoxifies, supports and restores optimum liver function through a rigorous programme that includes coffee enemas, enzyme therapy delivered through freshly juiced organic vegetables plus daily injections of vitamin B_{12} and liver extract. This programme is tough. It is not for everyone and it is not a miracle cure – the scientific evaluation of the programme is mixed and, when it does work, nobody can explain why. My argument is simply that everyone who has to make choices about cancer, for themselves or with a family member, should at least know about it.

The second treatment we all should at least have heard of goes by the name of the Essiac herbal formula. Essiac is *Caisse* backwards, which is the name of the Canadian nurse who devoted her life to testing this formula and bringing it to the attention of both patients and their doctors.

In the early 1920s, Rene Caisse was given a mysterious herbal formula by a patient who had successfully been treated for breast cancer by a Native American shamanic healer. Caisse, who went on to treat patients under the auspices of doctors and their clinics, claimed an 80% recovery rate but, to the day of her death in 1978, never divulged the exact formula she used.

The formula contains just four herbs – burdock, which is an excellent immune strengthener and which has been shown to have anti-tumour properties; sheep sorrel, which is believed to help reduce radiation damage and strengthen cell walls; a plant called turkey rhubarb, which cleanses the liver and again has an anti-tumour action, and slippery elm, which disperses swelling and supports the liver, spleen and pancreas.

You can brew these herbs into a tea to take twice a day, on an empty stomach, or buy ready-made liquid formulas which take the hassle out of making your own remedy. Tina Cooke, breast cancer survivor and founder of the UK's Cancer Alternative Information Bureau (CAIB), swears by this remedy and says, without it, she would not have survived.

Although there are scant clinical trials for the efficacy of this formula, the anecdotal evidence from people like Tina is overwhelming. Sadly there are many claims and counter-claims about the nature of the 'true' formula and who now owns it. My favourite observation on the whole subject, however, comes from an ancient medicine man practising in LA who, when asked about all the bickering over rights which followed Caisse's death, simply said: 'This formula is a gift from the Ojibwa to all mankind, all races, anyone! Why can't everyone just say thank you and accept it?'

(The Ojibwa were medicine men from Ontario. For a list of cancer support groups, see Resources.)

Candida Infection

Candida albicans is a yeast that lives chiefly in the bowel of almost every man, woman and child. Scientists have found no good reason for it to be there, but it does no harm either – until our immune system becomes compromised and allows it to multiply out of control.

Once this happens, the toxins it carries can interfere with almost every bodily function, and while you will not be at death's door, you certainly will not feel well. More common in women than men, chronic candidiasis has now been linked with recurring vaginal thrush and, in both sexes, with arthritis, autism, asthma, psoriasis and even infertility.

Poor co-ordination, muscle weakness, swollen or painful joints, mood swings, loss of libido, depression and unexplained tiredness can all be signs of infection by this organism, which will, if left unchecked, cause both digestive and hormonal disturbances. Insomnia, frequent ear, nose and throat infections and migraine-type headaches have also been reported by those subsequently found to be suffering severe yeast infections. It has even been linked with ME.

To tackle the root cause you need to support the immune system (see page 166), which, in most cases, has been weakened by either prolonged stress, illness or the over-prescribing of antibiotics. The latter, as we have seen, have an adverse effect because they wipe out the beneficial bacteria in the gut which co-exist with candida and, in optimum health, keep it in check. For women, taking the contraceptive pill can also trigger an infection.

If you think you may have this condition – and an estimated one-third of the population in the West is believed to have candida in one form or another – do a mental re-cap of your diet over the past week. The damp climate in the UK, for example, and underlying nutritional deficiencies, especially of zinc and the anti-stress B vitamins, all play a role in encouraging an overgrowth of yeast, but the biggest culprits are the dietary carbohydrates and sugars which the organism thrives on. Your first step, then, in bringing the infection back under control is to cut these foods from your diet.

Three times more common in women who wear nylon underwear or tights, it also makes sense to change to cotton fabrics. While in most cases sexual transmission is not an issue, if the infection persists it is worth getting both partners checked out.

To clear an infection, you need to first starve the organism of the fermented and sugary foods it thrives on. Cut out sugar-rich soft drinks and fruit juices, moderate your intake of tea, coffee and diet drinks and aim, instead, for eight glasses of pure water a day.

After a few weeks on your candida-elimination diet, you will then be ready to introduce herbs to boost the immune system and help clear the infection from the gut. Garlic, for example, is a potent antifungal agent with a strong anti-yeast action. It inhibits the growth of candida and has also been shown to help prevent recurring infections when taken over the long term. If you cannot face the idea of chewing a clove of garlic a day, look for odourless capsules, which provide 900mg per day of the active ingredient (allicin). Alternatively, take a fast-acting tincture. Aloe vera juice will also heal the damaged gut lining. Drink a quarter of a glass, twice a day.

The big anti-yeast herb is a little-known one called *pau d'arco* by the Portuguese, or *lapacho* by the Spanish-speaking population. It comes from South America where it is prized as a cure-all herb, and is taken from the inner bark of a native evergreen tree. When taken as a tea, it can help kill off the candida overgrowth – but it is a very potent herb and, in large quantities, should only be used under the supervision of a qualified health practitioner.

Your final attack to rid the body of a candida overgrowth for good will be to take a supplement to replace the so-called friendly bacteria in the digestive tract which will keep the candida that is present under control. Lots of people have now heard of probiotics but remain uncertain about why they need to take them or which brands to buy. Before making your choice, see page 171.

Caprylic acid, an extract from coconuts which has proved effective in keeping candida under control, is now frequently included in anti-candida supplements with great names such as Yeast Raiders. It beats taking pot luck with a topical application of live yoghurt and, according to tests by researchers at the East-West Clinic in Minnesota, it was voted by sufferers as best overall anti-candida treatment.

Anti-Candida Diet – At A Glance Guidelines

    Foods to eat: vegetables, nuts, seeds and oils
    Foods to moderate: whole grains, brown rice, oats and barley
    Foods to avoid: sugar, packaged and processed foods, yeast breads
    and pastries, mushrooms and truffles, most condiments and sauces,
    fruits (for the first three weeks of your candida-elimination diet) and
    re-heated leftovers.

Make sure any mineral and vitamin supplements you take are all yeast-free. Herbs are as potent as any prescription drugs – high doses of pau d'arco, for example, can cause bleeding, nausea and vomiting. Herbs can also interfere with existing medication, so seek advice from a qualified holistic health practitioner.

Cervical Smear Tests

If the results of a cervical smear test show the development of what are called 'abnormal' cells, then while it is important to make sure you go for your follow-up colposcopy examination, there is also a lot you can do with your diet to bolster your defences and help protect the cells from cancerous changes in the meantime. For example, women who eat selenium-rich broccoli at least three times a week have been shown to have an almost non-existent risk of suffering from cervical cancer. Introduce this into your diet, and also eat Brazil nuts to boost your selenium intake further.

Magnesium can protect the cell's membrane from cancer, which means you should be eating lots of magnesium-rich green, leafy vegetables, plus fruits, nuts and seeds. At the same time, cut down on the dairy in your diet, which has an adverse effect on magnesium levels.

You will already know that folic acid can help protect an unborn baby against neural tube defects and conditions such as Spina Bifida but you may not know it can help protect against cancerous changes to the cells of the cervix too. It will not be effective without adequate levels of vitamins B_{12}, B_3 and zinc so you need to take a good B vitamin complex rather than folic acid on its own.

If your smear test has already detected abnormal cervical cells, step up your vitamin C intake to 1g a day. You also need to make sure you are getting the right fats in your diet – especially the essential fatty acids (EFAs), which keep the cell membranes healthy. Eat oily fish and make sure you eat and cook with cold-pressed oils such as flax (linseed) and sunflower, from health food stores.

Cholesterol

High cholesterol is not an automatic death sentence. Up to a third of all those with a high cholesterol count never go on to develop either strokes or heart disease. Of course, that means two-thirds of this group do develop cardiovascular problems, but these can be avoided if changes to diet and lifestyle are introduced. Smoking, for example, must go.

Low thyroid function is one of the more common but often overlooked causes of high blood cholesterol. Rule this out by asking your doctor for a simple blood test. If there is a family history of this problem you may be more at risk, but again, you can swing the odds in your favour by adopting a healthy diet and lifesyle. As with so many common complaints, the root cause may be linked to impaired bowel function. A qualified nutritionist or naturopath will quickly determine whether this is a factor.

As well as measuring your so-called 'good cholesterol' or higher density lipoprotein (HDL) levels, ask your doctor to check your homocysteine levels. This is a normal byproduct of metabolism, which has been shown to be 40 times more accurate as an indicator of the risk of heart disease than cholesterol.

Cholesterol has a bad name, but we would not be alive without it. All the sex hormones, for example, are produced from cholesterol. In fact, medical students learn that the majority of the cholesterol in your body is made by the body itself. It is true, though, that cholesterol levels are raised more by saturated fats than any other food, so those big English and American-style breakfasts will have to stop. Instead, start your day with an oatbran porridge. Studies have shown that just 2–3oz of porridge a day can lower cholesterol levels by up to 10%. I make mine with water and have it throughout the winter.

Cholesterol-lowering drugs will obviously do the same job, but can have an adverse effect on the liver. It makes sense to investigate a more holistic approach using cholesterol-lowering herbs and vitamins including niacin or vitamin B_3. (Take a form of niacin such as Inositol that does not cause flushed skin.If you do feel flushed, it will pass after 20 minutes and should be relieved if you drink a glass of water.)

Garlic helps prevent heart disease by reducing blood pressure and blood lipids. Vitamin C reduces cholesterol; one of the richest sources are rosehips, which also contain bioflavonoids and other enzymes to enhance its action. Another less well-known but highly effective cholesterol-lowering agent is olive leaf extract. Oily fish and fresh, raw nuts (except peanuts) are excellent sources of the essential fatty acids which help to reduce blood pressure and keep the arteries elastic. Vitamin E 'thins' the blood, which takes pressure off the arteries – but do not take this as a supplement without supervision if you are already taking anti-coagulant prescription drugs which do the same job. Do not stop cholesterol-lowering medication without consulting your physician.

Protect the liver and lower cholesterol by sprinkling lethicin granules over your food. This works in the same way as HDL (which is made up mostly of lethicin) to protect the arteries. Lethicin has a detergent action that breaks up cholesterol in the body.

You can buy all these nutrients from health shops, of course, but one of the best cholesterol-lowering herbs is absolutely free. Dandelions, which are despised for being weeds, are an excellent natural source of lethicin. It is safe to eat the young leaves, which will make for an interesting side-salad.

Chronic Fatigue

The medical profession may continue to be divided about whether this condition even exists – it was only officially recognised in 1996 – but for those who suffer from it there is no doubt that Chronic Fatigue Syndrome is a debilitating illness which can ruin previously happy and fulfilled lives. There are no tests to confirm a diagnosis, although 60% of sufferers will have a specific protein in their blood called viral protein 1 (VP1).

The symptoms, which may include a sore throat, persistent infections, swollen lymph nodes, headaches, pain in the joints and muscles, depression, loss of appetite and a lack of concentration, are all totally debilitating. It should not, though, be confused with persistent fatigue or Tired All The Time syndrome (TATT), which affects an estimated 25% of the adult population.

To treat Chronic Fatigue, which tends to strike otherwise fit and healthy people and, among these, a higher than normal percentage of over-achievers, you need to understand and unravel the chain of events that has left sufferers with weakened immunity, impaired digestion, food allergies and aching limbs.

Prolonged stress, which keeps the body in a constant and heightened 'fight or flight' state, is the key culprit because, if allowed to go on, it will eventually compromise adrenal function. The adrenals are the glands that sit near the top of each kidney. The inner part (the medulla) secretes hormones, including adrenaline, that control blood pressure, heart rate and sweating. Under- or overproduction of any of the adrenal hormones can lead to serious illness.

Keeping the body under stress also lowers immunity, so when a virus does come along you are less able to resist it. Impaired immunity will adversely affect the digestive system. So will a viral attack, which will alter the balance of the microflora in the gut, setting up a condition called dysbiosis (see page 140) which prevents food from being properly digested, allows fermentation and irritates the lining of the gut. Once this starts, increased food sensitivities and even food allergies, which have been identified in 85% of dysbiosis sufferers, are almost inevitable. To remedy the problem, take a good probiotic (see page 171).

Food molecules which would not normally pass through an undamaged gut lining trigger an allergic reaction when this damage allows them to penetrate. They are seen as marauding invaders by the immune system, which becomes even more undermined by these ongoing challenges. You are then ripe for a serious candida infection (see page 109).

If you feel worn out just reading about this vicious cycle of events, imagine what state your body will be in having to fight it. Naturopaths, who treat disease with natural remedies including nutrition, homeopathy and herbalism but who avoid allopathic drugs, take the view that Chronic Fatigue, Fibromyalgia and Myalgic Encephalomyelitis (ME) present such similar symptoms that they will benefit from the same treatment plan.

Increasingly, this will include liquorice. More traditionally used for gastric problems, especially ulcers, its resurgence as a treatment for fatigue was sparked by a letter in the *New Zealand Medical Journal* from an Italian physician who reportedly cured his own Chronic Fatigue by taking about 4g per day.

Liquorice acts on the blood pressure and so ties in with one of the latest theories about the underlying causes of Chronic Fatigue. The suggestion, based on limited tests, is that following an initial viral infection, sufferers are left with an inability to regulate their blood pressure. One American study, for example, found that at the exact point where the heart rate would need to speed up to cope with extra exertion, in those suffering from Chronic Fatigue, it actually slows down.

The active ingredient in liquorice is glycyrrhizinic acid – a plant steroid that mimics one of the prescription drugs given to treat this low blood pressure irregularity. Liquorice also enhances the action of corticosteroids, the hormones produced by the outer layer of the adrenal glands.

Another theory is that Chronic Fatigue is the body's desperate response to an overload of toxins. To remedy this, you should try a basic detox diet (see page 130) which eliminates wheat, dairy and meat from your diet for two weeks. Also, try and drink 2 litres of water daily to flush out toxins. Chronic fatigue has also now been linked with a deficiency of the B vitamins, and of minerals such as magnesium which may help relieve the muscular pain patients complain of.

This is the most difficult symptom of all to treat, but there is some hope on the horizon. Preliminary but uncontrolled trials have suggested a combination of higher doses of magnesium (600mg) and malic acid (2,400mg) can help. The latter is a naturally occurring organic acid which plays a critical role in the production of ATP – carrier of the energy that fuels the entire body.

For support groups to help with Chronic Fatigue, see Resources.

Cold Sores

The two main triggers of the herpes simplex 1 virus, which causes cold sores, are sunlight and stress. If you are a sufferer you need to start thinking about protecting yourself from an unsightly outbreak at about the same time you pack for your summer holiday or arrange your Christmas party.

The first line of defence is to boost your immune system (see page 166). Complementary health really comes into its own here, with a combination of herbal, homoeopathic and nutritional steps to suppress the virus (which cannot be destroyed outright) and keep it dormant.

Although a homoeopathic constitutional diagnosis is always better in the long term, if you are already on holiday and away from your homoeopath when a herpes outbreak threatens, it is wise to dose yourself homoeopathically and support the system while it is under attack. If you tend to get cold sores in the sun and they start with that familiar itchy tingle, take the homoeopathic remedy Natrum mur 30c. If an outbreak begins with more of a sharp, prickling pain and the sore tends to crack and bleed, you need to take homeopathic Nitric acid 30c.

The cold sore virus is activated by an amino acid called arginine. Another amino acid, called lysine, inhibits the absorption of arginine and therefore helps suppress this virus. Foods that are rich in arginine (and which you need to avoid) include chocolate, nuts and most cereal grains. Natural sources of lysine include dairy products, potatoes and brewer's yeast, so step up your dietary intake of these and take a lysine supplement too.

Zinc, which boosts the immune system, has also been shown to help. Food sources include oysters, seafood, eggs, liver, turkey, and sunflower and pumpkin seeds, but if you plan to take more than 30mg a day for several months, you will need to balance this with a copper supplement of 2mg a day. (Note – Patients diagnosed with Alzheimer's Disease should not take zinc supplements until researchers have clarified the role of this mineral in the disease.)

One of the most potent and less well-known antidotes to cold sores is St John's Wort – or nature's Prozac – which is more usually taken for mild to moderate depression. It has fantastic antiviral properties and, although reported side-effects include increased photosensitivity in sunlight, this has only been recorded among cows grazing on meadows of the herb, and not in humans.

 If you fail to suppress the virus and a cold sore does develop, grapefruit seed extract or Citricidal has strong antibacterial and antiviral properties and is safe to dab on the sore. Dabbing vaseline on the sore will prevent any recurrence on that site. If you suffer from recurrent sores, your immune system is compromised and needs supporting with herbs such as elderflower, astralagus or liquorice.

With cold sores, prevention is the key. I have heard strong anecdotal reports of a wonder supplement called Elagen, in which the active ingredient is an Asian plant called *Eleutherococcus senticosus* which is said to bolster the body's natural defences. After Trading Standards litigation in the UK, the manufacturer was forced to withdraw claims that it could help cure cancer, but the prosecuting lawyers did not dispute the suggestion that it is an effective immune enhancer – and as such, it works to keep the cold sore virus at bay.

Constipation

This is a problem which secretly blights the lives of millions of people, especially women, who suffer in silence and who think it is normal to empty their bowels only once every three days. A healthy colon will be emptying the bowel three times a day, usually after every meal, so you can use this to gauge the extent of your own problem.

One of the most important dietary factors in preventing constipation is eating the right kind of fibre, plus fruit, vegetables and plenty of water. The latter, especially, helps soften the stools, making them easier to pass through the digestive tract. Aim for eight glasses of unpolluted, still water every day.

The gluten in processed wheat is difficult for many adults to digest – if eating wheat causes your stomach to bloat, this can be a sign of a growing intolerance. Avoid both wheat and mucus-producing dairy products until your digestion is running smoothly again.

I wanted to call my first book (*The Vitality Cookbook*) the 'Poo Bible', but the publisher was not impressed! The fact is, when we spent a fortnight testing out the recipes, the whole household became as regular as clockwork, dutifully eliminating after every meal. Many of these recipes were designed to tackle constipation and the digestive disorders which now cause more days off work, after the common cold, than any other condition.

If you depend on laxatives for relief, you are making a big mistake. Far from solving the problem, they actually increase it by making the colon lazy. You need to re-educate your digestive tract. One of the gentlest ways to start this is to introduce psyllium seeds into your diet. These swell as they mop up fluid during their passage through the digestive tract, and so add bulk to the faeces. Take a tablespoon sprinkled on your cereal in the morning or on your salad at lunchtime. If you dislike the idea of seeds, which can irritate a damaged gut, you can also use flaxseed oil to counter constipation.

You may also be deficient in the so-called 'good bacteria' which aid digestion. Again, you can remedy this by taking a good probiotic (see page 171) to replenish levels of the organisms which help.

Insufficient gastric acidity is another cause. Remedy this by taking cider vinegar with meals.

Cystitis

Cystitis is an inflammation of the bladder and/or urethra, which is the tube through which urine passes from the bladder and out of the body. This inflammation is a result of infection, bruising or irritation. While the irritation and bruising can be caused by using barrier contraceptives, or may be the result of sexual intercourse, an infection is usually caused by the micro-organism *Escherichia coli* (*E. coli*) which will have travelled from the anus, via the urethra, to the bladder.

Far more common in women than in men (because of the close proximity of the urethra and the vagina to the anus), the symptoms – which may include burning pain on passing water, a dragging pain in the abdomen and lower back, an unpleasant smell to the urine (which may also contain blood) and a frequent urge to urinate – make life hell for thousands of sufferers. Many women suffer their first attack around the time of menopause, when a reduction in levels of the female hormone, oestrogen, causes a thinning of the tissues of the urethra and the vagina.

One good reason to seek out an alternative remedy is that between 50 and 80% of all the bacteria in the body are resistant to conventional treatment, and cystitis, which often flares up during pregnancy, can even be *caused* by prescription drugs.

Cranberries are the best known of the natural remedies. They contain a substance called hippuric acid which prevents the *E. coli* bacteria from sticking to the walls of the bladder. Cranberry juice also changes the acidity of the urine, to stop the bacteria from multiplying. It is important you buy a non-sweetened brand. Aim to drink 16 fl oz a day. If you cannot face this, take cranberry in supplement form. Drinking 2 litres of pure water flavoured with fresh lime daily will also help prevent re-infection.

On the subject of whether the urine should be acidified or alkalised to best treat cystitis, complementary practitioners are divided, although most now seem to promote the idea that it is better to raise the pH and make the urine more alkaline, which is actually easier than making it more acidic. At the first signs of an attack, dissolve a teaspoon of bicarbonate of soda in water and drink, three times a day, until the infection has passed.

In traditional Ayurvedic medicine, which treats patients according to their constitutional type (see page 272), the remedy for cystitis includes some 23 different herbs. A simpler Ayurvedic-based remedy is to boil 4 tablespoons of antibacterial coriander seeds in 4 cups of water until the liquid reduces by half. Strain and mix with a little honey to drink.

Although you should avoid chemical irritants including soaps, bubble baths and bath oils during an attack, you can use the antiseptic essential oils to help soothe the inflammation. Bergamot has an affinity with the genito-urinary system and is also excellent for thrush and vaginal itching. Dilute and mix with antiseptic lavender and sandalwood, which is also highly effective against cystitis, in your bath.

Bioflavanoids are responsible for the colour of the leaves, flowers and stems of food plants and many of the medicinally active ingredients in herbs are bioflavanoids. Once known as vitamin P, they have excellent anti-inflammatory properties and work best when eaten with vitamin C. Best natural sources include citrus fruits, apricots, cherries, green peppers and broccoli. The richest source of all is the central white core of citrus fruits. Other recommended dietary changes include avoiding all sugars and refined carbohydrates, diluting fruit juices and cutting down on known food allergens such as wheat and dairy products.

Another less well-known herb which will help tackle cystitis and prevent reinfection is Uva ursi or bearberry (*Arctostaphylos uva-ursi*). A small, evergreen shrub, which grows on moors and mountains, the leaves act as a urinary antiseptic thanks to a chemical called arbutin. In the body, this is converted to *hydroquinone*, a related compound with known urinary tract antiseptic properties. Uva ursi is said to be particularly effective against *E. coli* – but again, it works better when the urine is diluted, so drink plenty of pure water. Uva ursi tablets are available but only on prescription from your healthcare practitioner.

In one double-blind study of 57 women, none of the 30 women given standardised Uva ursi extract had a recurrence of bladder infection at the end of 12 months. Of the 27 women given a placebo, five suffered re-infection. Neither group reported any side-effects, although if taken in excess Uva ursi can cause unpleasant reactions including nausea, vomiting and shortness of breath. The best way to take this herb is in tincture form or as a tea, but it should be avoided during pregnancy.

Juicing will also help. In his book *SuperJuice*, the UK naturopath and broadcaster Michael van Straten suggests a delicious Pink Punch cocktail of cranberries, strawberries, stoned cherries and pink grapefruit to help fight off the bacteria that cause cystitis. While the cranberries help prevent the infection, the juice is also rich in vitamin C to boost immunity and help the whole body fight back to good health. To make van Straten's Pink Punch juice, mix 1 peeled and pithed pink grapefruit, 6oz stoned cherries, 6oz cranberries and 6oz strawberries.

Finally, take 1,000mg of vitamin C every day and, when you do have an attack, dissolve 1 teaspoon of echinacea tincture in apple juice or water and take this twice a day until the infection is over.

Deodorants

Scientists are currently investigating suggestions of a link between the use of deodorants, particularly anti-perspirants, and breast cancer rates in women.

The theory, to date clinically unproven, is that chemicals called *parabens*, which are used as preservatives in deodorants, could be responsible for accelerating the growth of tumours in the breast.

Dismissed as nothing more than scaremongering by august groups such as The American Cancer Society and the UK's Cancer Research Campaign, the theory gained credence because what scientists do know is that a woman is eight times more likely to develop breast cancer in that area of the breast closest to the underarm than in any other part of the breast tissue.

Most doctors believe the link to deodorants is no more than an unfortunate health myth, but if you are concerned (and one of the British researchers now examining tumour tissue from thousands of breast cancer patients is worried enough to have stopped using anti-perspirants herself) there are several, more natural alternatives.

The problem with many commercial deodorants is that they contain aluminium compounds – particularly Aluminium chlorohydrate – which are easily absorbed through the skin and which have, in the only reported trial to date, already been linked with higher risks of Alzheimer's.

If you want to take the totally natural route, you can use salt crystals to deodorise armpits. These are available from most health stores (see Resources).

Dr Andrew Weil, the US holistic health guru, says that rubbing alcohol (which acts as an antibacterial agent) onto the skin will work, but if you don't want to step out of the house whiffing of vodka (and as a teetotaller I, for one, don't) then try one of the more natural roll-on deodorants instead. I like the Nature's

Gate product, which contains an oak-derived odour-eater, sage, myrrh and witch hazel, but then I don't mind smelling of incense. A more popular brand is Tom's of Maine, which comes in Aloe & Coriander, or All Scents and which gets the thumbs up from authors of *The Safe Shopper's Bible*.

Depression

In Germany, doctors treating depression now prescribe the herbal remedy, St John's Wort, 10 times more often than its orthodox cousin, Prozac. There are numerous clinical studies showing how, for the treatment of mild to moderate depression, it is as effective as any of the conventional antidepressants with the added bonus of fewer side-effects.

In recent placebo-controlled trials reported in the *British Medical Journal*, German researchers found, for example, that a daily dose of 900 micrograms of hypericin, one of the active ingredients in the herb, was as effective as 100mg of the orthodox antidepressant, imipramine, in improving the quality of life for sufferers. They also found that because patients can tolerate St John's Wort better than most of the tricyclic antidepressants, they are more likely to keep taking it.

Cattle grazing on large quantities of the herb have shown increased photosensitivity, but this reaction has not been recorded in humans. What is more of a problem is the fact St John's Wort has prescription-only status in a number of European countries and that, under proposed EC guidelines, this number is growing.

If you are resident in one of those countries where you cannot buy St John's Wort over the counter, you should investigate a less well-known supplement. SAMe, pronounced *Sammy*, is now prescribed for depression in 14 different countries. It has proved so popular since its launch in the US in the Spring of 1999 that it now ranks 25th among the 13,000 supplements currently on sale in health stores.

SAMe – short for S-adenosylmethionine – is neither herb, vitamin nor hormone. It is a molecule produced by all living cells which, like so many new supplements, is said to be vital to the health of all the body's tissues and organs. Levels decline with age – kids have seven times more SAMe than adults – and it is now believed to play an important role in the regulation of neurotransmitters, especially those controlling mood.

The way it works is through a process called *methylation*, which occurs naturally a billion times a second throughout the body, affecting every biological system from the development of the foetus to the basic maintenance of cell membranes. Methylation describes a simple chemical transaction in which a molecule donates a four-atom appendage (a methyl group) to an adjacent molecule. Both molecules then change shape. Biochemists stress the importance of methylation by claiming that without it there would be no life as we know it. Lots of molecules can do this, but of all the identified methyl donors, SAMe is said to be the most active.

The body makes its own SAMe from methionine, an amino acid provided in protein-rich foods, but once it has lost its methyl group it is then broken down to form homocysteine. This potentially harmful (in excess) waste product, circulated in the bloodstream, has been identified as a powerful predictor of the risk of heart disease – some 40 times more accurate than cholesterol levels –

and so this is *not* something you want to leave swishing around your body to build up in your cells.

To avoid this, you keep your homocysteine levels low by making sure the body has enough vitamin B_6, B_{12} and folic acid (found in fruits and vegetables) which then re-convert the offending substance back to glusathione, said to be the most potent anti-cancer agent in the body and a powerful antioxidant used in its own right to eliminate the free radical toxins caused by smoking and drinking. B vitamin deficiencies are common in both sexes, but research shows some 20% of those patients hospitalised due to depression are seriously lacking in vitamin B_6. The body cannot store any of the B vitamins, which are also wiped out by prescription drugs, the contraceptive pill, alcohol and too much sugar and coffee. Low levels of vitamin B_{12} are also known to trigger depression.

SAMe is thought to help by enhancing the impact of the mood-lifting brain chemicals serotonin and dopamine. It is not known whether it does this by regulating the biochemistry and breakdown of these substances or by making the receptor sites they latch on to in the brain even more responsive. The clinical evidence for SAMe is small but persuasive – just 40 clinical trials involving 1,400 patients since the 1970s – and while nobody is claiming this molecule is more effective than the conventional drug treatments, it has been shown to be less toxic, with a mild stomach ache likely to be the only side-effect. If you are taking conventional treatments, do not stop and switch to SAMe without medical consultation and supervision. If, however, your depression is mild and you would benefit from a mood-booster, SAMe could work for you.

Another natural remedy frequently used to treat the blues, especially in the winter in colder climates, is Kava Kava. A member of the pepper family, it contains kavalactones, which relax muscles and have a calming effect on the whole body and the mind. It is not addictive but there is a small risk you may feel drowsy when you first start taking it. If you do, avoid driving. I prefer to recommend this in tincture form since it gets into the bloodstream faster this way.

Of the natural antidepressants found in foods, an amino acid called phenylalanine is one of the best. You'll find this in chocolate and cheese. It is the substance the brain makes more of when you fall in love, so you can see why it might become addictive. It is sold in supplement form as DL-phenylalanine or DLPA, which boosts mood by restoring normal levels of endorphins. It can take two weeks to kick in, but once working you should only need to take it for a week in every month.

DeTox Diet

If you are not confident about embarking on any kind of serious detox plan, then consult your doctor or a qualified health practitioner who can hold your hand through the programme. One of my favourites is this one, devised by the talented holistic health practitioners and medical herbalists at Farmacia in London – the UK's first pharmacy with on-suite complementary therapies. These health therapists live and work in the very heart of the city and know how important it is to give the body a rest from the onslaught of environmental and dietary pollutants it has to deal with each and every day. It is a three-week DeTox and I like to do it at the end of winter when spring is in the air and when, in the countryside where I live, everything that has been in hibernation and storing its energy is stirring back into life.

Investing in a good quality juicer will make it easier to stick to this programme, but before you begin, empty the cupboards of all those tempting but unhealthy foods which are not good for you. Remove all foods containing wheat, dairy and sugar which are three of the biggest allergens responsible for food intolerances, and replace them instead with healthy rice noodles, vegetable soups, cereals, oatbran and rye breads.

To follow this plan, work with your digestive system by combining foods that will not fight in the gut. If, for example, you have starch for lunch, have protein for supper or vice versa, but avoid eating these two food groups together. Eat fruit on its own, at least half an hour before or after other foods, and try to eat a 50% raw diet, which will supply the enzymes crucial to digestion.

Try and drink 2 litres of fluid every day – this must not include tea, coffee or sugary soft drinks, all of which are banned. Drink water if you feel hungry between meals, and drink lots of herbal teas, especially camomile, fennel and peppermint, which all soothe and aid digestion.

The basic plan you are going to follow is:

Breakfast

Fresh fruit, oatmeal or a breakfast cereal which does not contain wheat or sugar, such as millet.

Lunch

Soup and/or salad with a carbohydrate such as oat cakes or rice cakes. Or you can have a protein and vegetable meal, say stir-fry of grains and vegetables.

Supper

Have either protein or starch (the opposite to your lunch), salad and/or a non-dairy homemade soup.

Mid-morning Snacks

Juiced vegetables and fruits; sunflower and pumpkin seeds, raw almonds and cashew nuts. Sesame tahini with rice cakes is a filling alternative. Soya yoghurts will boost the detox, and if you crave something starchy and sweet, make your own banana and raisin bread with soya flour.

Start each day with the so-called Master Cleanse Drink which combines 1 cup of water, the juice of half an organic lemon, a pinch of cayenne pepper and 2 tsp of honey, organic maple syrup or molasses. Heat gently to serve warm.

About 30 minutes before lunch, make the same drink again but add 1–2 tsp of finely grated ginger. This is another old Ayurvedic trick to stimulate the gastric juices and help digestion.

In the second week of this DeTox, take vitamin C and a good multivitamin to make sure your body is still getting all the nutrients it needs.

Warning

Any serious DeTox or cleansing programme can trigger what is called a healing crisis. This can range from a migraine-like headache to flu-type symptoms. Expect wild mood swings as your body adjusts to its new eating plan. Skin rashes, diarrhoea, bad breath, insomnia and increased sensitivity to cold are all additional signs of the body spring-cleaning itself and having a good flush-out of damaging toxins.

See also Fasting DeTox Diet, page 147.

Diarrhoea

Acute diarrhoea may be caused by an infection and may mean you need to see your doctor. You should definitely consult a health practitioner if it lasts for more than four days, since there may be a more serious underlying condition. Diarrhoea which alternates with constipation is a classic sign of a very common condition called Irritable Bowel Syndrome (IBS); to manage this, see page 178.

Too much coffee can cause diarrhoea in some people. Taking high doses (over 2g) of vitamin C can have the same side-effect, and drinking fruit juice, which is high in fructose (which holds on to water as it passes through the gut) can all be to blame. Cut these out for a few days and see if it makes any difference to your symptoms.

Simple food combining will help relieve diarrhoea. This means eating proteins such as meat, fish, cheese, eggs and nuts separately from carbohydrates such as bread, cereals, pasta, potatoes and rice. Acid-tasting fruits should be eaten with protein, not starch. Cakes, sweets, biscuits, chocolate, coffee, fatty or fried foods and fizzy drinks should be eliminated altogether. Ripe papaya and pineapple both contain digestive enzymes that will help restore normal functioning; both are available in supplement form.

The Chinese favour a tea made from germinated barley, called *mai ya* which you can buy from Chinese herb suppliers (see Resources). It sounds horrible but drinking rice water – made by boiling and mashing rice and then straining off the water – will also combat diarrhoea.

To relax and tone the bowel, herbalists recommend drinking equal parts of fennel, agrimony, camomile and mint. The essential oils in this brew are antispasmodic, and agrimony is a gentle astringent which will encourage more solid stools.

Acute diarrhoea can damage the gut lining. Aloe vera juice (a quarter of a glass, twice a day) or large doses of folic acid (5,000mcg, three times a day) can help repair this.

An attack of diarrhoea can leave you with a deficiency in vitamins and minerals which the body has not been able to absorb, especially vitamin A and zinc. To counter this, take a good multisupplement. If you have had diarrhoea, it also makes sense to replenish levels of the good gut bacteria that have been wiped out, with a probiotic supplement.

Dietary Cleansing

You may think your diet is healthy and that you are looking after your health, but scientists have discovered that, on average, the number of E-coded chemicals and artificial flavourings we consume in our food adds up to the equivalent of 18 tablets of soluble aspirin every day. Most of us digest a staggering 3,000 chemicals every day. Current testing methods cannot detect more than half the chemicals known to be used in food production, and there are no tests at all for what happens when these chemicals or other additives find their way into the body via the food chain and then combine together or get broken down to form new substances called metabolites, which may be harmful. Remember, of the produce in your supermarket, less than 1% has been tested for such pollutants anyway.

Think about how cigarette smoke, a known carcinogen and pollutant, irritates the eyes, throat and nostrils of the non-smoker or the person trying to smoke for the first time. Then ask yourself how these other additives and chemicals in the foods we eat might just have a similar effect on the tissues inside the body.

In my research into how diet and nutrition play a role in many degenerative diseases – ranging from rheumatism and arthritis to kidney problems and a condition called sarcoidosis – I have been introduced to a very effective cleansing diet first championed in the 1930s and resurrected by the doctors at the UK-based Good HealthKeeping group.

The theory, which was first supported by Benedict Lust, the founding father of naturopathy, is that acidic material, left over after the digestion of protein in the liver, builds up in the blood where it forms loose 'globules' of more concentrated acid. These then disturb normal metabolism and settle around the joints. At first, they are semi-solid and relatively easy to reabsorb back into the bloodstream for disposal, but over time they solidify, causing the inflammation responsible for some 200 different types of arthritis. The diet that helped prevent this was devised by a Dr Max Bircher-Benner, working with bedridden arthritis patients in the 1930s. It has been further refined to become a mucus-less diet too. While designed specifically for muscular-skeletal conditions, this diet is just as effective if you simply want to boost energy levels by giving your body a rest from toxins in food.

The Diet

First, cut out sugar in all its form. Check food labels for hidden sugar content. Eliminate white or refined flour. Stick to wholemeal and avoid coffee, strong Indian tea, cola drinks and chocolate.

Start your cleansing diet with a two-day fast, drinking only home-made barley water or mineral or filtered tap water. This is likely to provoke what is known as a healing crisis: you may feel as if you have all the symptoms of flu, so it is probably wise to embark on this when you have time off work. Your body is actually undergoing a spring-clean, which can be unnerving, so make sure, before you start, that you have the support of a qualified health practitioner or your doctor to see you through this.

After these first two days, you can begin to eat one or two pieces of fresh fruit at your normal mealtimes. For variety, alternate with raw vegetables. When you feel well and hungry again, have just two meals a day. Have a late breakfast or lunch and then an evening meal. Drink lemon barley water between meals, but do not drink with food or for an hour after you have eaten.

For Breakfast

Start the day with a cup of juniper berry tea, brewed overnight. Eat a generous fresh fruit course and eat as much as you like. Add mixed nuts and raisins and, if you are still hungry, have dry wholemeal toast.

For Your Main Meal

Make a generous fresh coleslaw of cabbage, onion and carrot, and start with this. Use only organic vegetables. Have a short break and then eat a baked vegetable; try potatoes, broccoli or cauliflower. Cook your vegetables slowly and gently in their own juices and in a covered dish.

Follow this cleansing diet for three weeks, then return to a more normal diet but keep off those foods you (and your body) now recognise as being unwholesome.

If you suffer from rheumatoid arthritis, this cure will take months, not weeks. Carry on avoiding all meat, fish, shellfish, tinned food, eggs, spices, salt, coffee, Indian tea, alcohol and tobacco. You may include a little butter and cottage cheese but should avoid all other dairy products.

Supplement your cleansing diet with zinc, vitamin C and vitamin B complex. This regimen is also fantastic for shifting that small but persistent amount of weight you never seem to be able to lose, and for reducing water retention. It can also be helpful in treating the so-called auto-immune conditions such as sarcoidosis (see page 221) and IgA nephropathy. If you suffer from these, immune-supporting herbs such as echinacea, Siberian ginseng and aloe vera will also help.

Warning

This is a rigorous cleansing diet. If you have any underlying medical complaint, do not embark on it without medical supervision.

Diverticular Disease

Diverticular disease is the general term used to describe a number of different disorders that affect the intestinal tract. A diverticulum is a sac-like pouch found on any part of the gastrointestinal tract but most common, by far, in the large intestine, especially along the last section, just before the rectum. The presence of these pouches is called *diverticulosis*, which frequently develops after middle age. If the diverticula become inflamed, which usually only happens when food becomes trapped in a pouch, then the condition is known as diverticulitis.

Diverticulosis is said to have no symptoms, but disruptions to the digestive system, including painful cramps, diarrhoea and constipation, have all been linked to the problem. Severe abdominal pain and fever are all signs of diverticulitis. A liquid diet, rest and antibiotics are usually prescribed for mild cases of this disease, but some 20% of sufferers do not improve and are subsequently operated on. Of those under the age of 50 who do need surgery, men outnumber women three to one.

David Crawford is a UK nutritionist who specialises in using natural foods to treat such problems. He says it is correct that you need a high-fibre diet (this is what most sufferers are told), but stresses there is an even greater risk to your health if you eat the wrong type of fibre. You need, for example, to avoid all the mucus-forming grains, including wheat, rye and dairy, since these will exacerbate the problem. Instead, look for fibre from chickpea or soya flours, from fruit and vegetables and from oatbran and sprouted grains.

Diverticular disease is usually the result of prolonged constipation, caused by a long, slow build-up of dietary mucus against the walls of the intestine. Over time, these deposits solidify, narrowing the passage through which the faeces must pass. The intestine responds by trying to expand to maintain normal functioning, and it is in the weakened areas of the intestinal walls that the first diverticular pouches appear. A clever nutritionist will know how you can dissolve this build-up of waste matter without resorting to more invasive techniques such as colonic irrigation, where, if the intestinal wall has been damaged, there could be further risks.

David Crawford's treatment plan for this condition, for example, includes a tailor-made juicing regimen, likely to include carrot and apple juice in the mornings, carrot and celery in the evenings and a combination of carrot, beetroot and cucumber in between times. An excellent tip for maintaining good digestive health for everyone is to drink a cup of warm water with the juice of half a lemon when you get up in the mornings.

If you are suffering the milder symptoms of this disease, avoid nuts and seeds, which can irritate and get trapped in the diverticulae. Instead, eat more pineapple and papaya, both of which contain potent digestive enzymes that will help reduce inflammation. This is one condition where it is crucial to treat the underlying cause. Psyllium husks, which make up the branded fibre products which are often recommended, can help alleviate the symptoms but do not attack the cause. If left untreated, these conditions can lead to more serious, even carcinogenic, conditions. This is because, after digestion, the residue of bile salts can react with any putrefying food (especially meat) that has become trapped in the pouches, to create cancer-causing metabolites. This is a risk, not an unavoidable prognosis, but it highlights the importance of tackling the root cause of any digestive disturbance.

Dysbiosis

In a recent survey by The Industrial Society, digestive disorders were cited as the second most common cause of absenteeism, after the common cold. For those who suffer the embarrassment of them, this is no joke. For example, Irritable Bowel Syndrome (IBS), which affects an estimated 20% of the adult population and twice as many women as men, causes alternating constipation and diarrhoea, making it difficult for sufferers to cope away from the home and especially at work.

Keeping the digestion healthy should be as simple as eating a high-fibre diet, drinking plenty of water and maintaining a healthy balance of the microflora in the gut. Clearly, however, many people are struggling both to digest and eliminate their food – a process which uses up 80% of our energy – properly.

Naturopaths – those complementary health practitioners who treat illness without resorting to allopathic drugs – now suggest that 70% of all diseases are caused, initially, by problems with digestion. And the most common disorder is one you probably don't even know you have.

Dysbiosis is the term used to describe an imbalance of the bacteria in the digestive tract. In a healthy gut, you would expect to find around 3 pounds of bacteria, with the so-called 'friendly' ones making up a third of the population at best. At worst, and especially after the prolonged use of antibiotics or years of a diet that is too high in saturated fats, refined foods and sugar, levels of the good bacteria may be so low that they are virtually undetectable.

Conditions linked with dysbiosis include IBS, acne, food allergies, Chronic Fatigue and depression. You can help repopulate the good bacteria by eating foods that act as natural probiotics. These include bananas, artichokes, asparagus and honey. But for real impact, you need to take a probiotic supplement (see page 171) and Fructo-oligosaccharides (FOS), a sweet-tasting powder, which acts as a 'fast food' for these health-promoting bacteria.

Eczema

Worldwide, eczema is now three times more common than asthma. In the UK it affects some 4% of the under-12s. Researchers believe the problem is a genetic one, exacerbated by environmental pollutants, but diet also plays a role. Sufferers have been found, for example, to be unable to digest a protein found in milk called casein. So changing the diet to cut out dairy products should help. If you are worried about your calcium intake, you probably can digest the casein in both sheep and goats' products, so switch to these. Refined sugar in food will also make your eczema worse, so start reading food labels and avoid it like the plague!

Rosa mosqueta (rosehip) oil has been formulated specifically for scar tissue (it is also excellent on wrinkles) and will help reduce the lividity of any residual scar tissue. For suppliers, see Resources and then simply massage it into the affected areas every day.

Sandra Gibbons, holistic skin and Dead Sea treatment specialist (see Resources) also recommends a bath emollient called Aveeno oatmeal and a skin gel called Witch Doctor gel, both of which will help soothe the irritation. A psoriasis sufferer who has now been 'clear' for 25 years, she has spent years investigating the value of the healing powers of the mineral-rich Dead Sea, and has now established the Dead Sea Therapy Centre in London, which is getting good results with both eczema and psoriasis. She reports that the salinity of the Dead Sea on the Jordanian side is 27% (on the Israeli shore it is 37%), and therefore milder for wet eczema and sore and broken skin. Patients exposed to the less intense, more effectively filtered sunlight on both shores report an enviable 85% recovery rate too.

Stephen Terrass, another holistic health expert who is currently technical director with Solgar vitamins UK and the author of *Eczema & Psoriasis*, also cleared his own severe eczema with an alternative programme that started by eliminating the two main culprits in food intolerance – wheat and dairy. He suggests you also take a good multivitamin supplement which is rich in the antioxidant vitamins A and E, plus a high dose of zinc (40–50mg) per day.

Staphylococcus aureus, one of the so-called Superbugs which is resistant to the most commonly-used antibiotics, has been implicated in exacerbating and spreading eczema in the majority of cases, so you will need to boost your holistic eczema treatment with a strong antibacterial agent. Choose from goldenseal, echinacea or burdock, all herbs which will strengthen your immune system. You can take these internally, or, for a soothing antibacterial facewash, infuse your chosen herb in a pint of boiling water. Allow to cool. Filter through a coffee filter paper and splash over the affected area.

Lots of sufferers have also found relief with quercetin – an anti-allergenic flavanoid found naturally but in small quanities in red cherries, onions, garlic, broccoli and cauliflower. It has excellent anti-inflammatory properties and has now become one of the biggest-selling supplements in the US.

Starflower cream can relieve the itching, especially in children. As well as borage, it contains camomile and chickweed, both of which can treat many other skin conditions too. Napiers, for example, make an Infant starflower which can be used for children over four months old and which is also very good for irritated facial skin in adults.

One of my best discoveries is SK Cream made by British organic farmers David and Margaret Evans in their old cow barn in Lincolnshire. I heard about it from a nursery nurse who wrote saying she always keeps a jar close by for small children who are having problems with their eczema. The makers never advertise this cream, but ship thousands of jars all over the world thanks to this kind of word-of-mouth recommendation. Keep it in the fridge and, if you are allergic to preservatives, get the version that is lanolin-free (see Resources).

Endometriosis

This is a very painful condition where the same sort of cells that grow in the lining of the womb begin to grow outside the uterus. One theory is that these cells actually migrate from the uterus. Another is that they are different types of cells that have mutated due to an error in their genetic programming.

The most likely sites for endometriosis to occur are the ovaries, the Fallopian tubes, the bladder and the bowel. Symptoms range from painful periods to infertility and, in many cases, major surgery is undertaken. High levels of the female hormone, oestrogen, are common in women with endometriosis, so your first step should be to try and normalise these. The B vitamins play an important role here because they generate the liver enzymes that convert oestrogen in the form of oestradiol – which causes these cells to proliferate, into a safer form called oestriol, which can be excreted.

The reason endometriosis is so painful is that it is an inflammatory condition. Essential fatty acids (EFAs) can counter this by producing substances called prostaglandins, which have a natural anti-inflammatory action. The best source is an unpolluted fish or evening primrose oil. Many sufferers have low levels of zinc, which also has a potent inflammatory action, so take at least 15mg a day.

DL-phenylalanine (DLPA) is a natural painkiller. It works in 60% of those who take it, but takes several weeks to take effect. If you see no improvement after three weeks, it is not the solution for you. When it does work, the theory is that it promotes the production of endorphins – the body's own, natural painkillers – and interferes with the brain's perception of pain by altering the action of the neurotransmitters (chemical messengers). Do not take DLPA if pregnant, breast-feeding, taking antidepressants or if you have high blood pressure.

A qualified herbalist can also help using hormonal balancing herbs such as agnus castus, false unicorn root and lady's mantle. Raspberry leaf is an important tonic for the whole reproductive system. When the pain is bad, herbs such as camomile, wild yam and blue cohosh can provide relief. Saw palmetto, which is used in preparations to support the prostate gland in men, can block the action of the sex hormone called Follicle Stimulating Hormone (FSH), which is known to increase endometrial tissue. However, with a condition this serious do not try and self-treat. Instead, find a practitioner who has treated it successfully before, and join a support group (see Resources).

Erectile Dysfunction

Inadequate blood flow to the penis is a major cause of erectile dysfunction. The herb most often prescribed for circulatory problems is Ginkgo biloba. In one study, reported in the medical journal *Urology*, 50 impotent men were given

240mg of Ginkgo biloba daily for nine months. Some of the men were also given papaverine, a muscle stimulant that can also help improve erections. The researchers reported that the Ginkgo biloba supplement greatly improved sexual performance in both groups, regardless of the papaverine.

Although there is a long tradition of using this herb for circulatory and sexual problems in Asia, science is only now beginning to explain how it works. Molecular biologists at the University of California, for example, believe Ginkgo's primary role in the body may be as a regulator of nitric oxide, which is critical for many body functions, including circulation.

Essential fatty acids are also crucial to sexual health. One of the best sources, for both men and women, is linseed (flaxseed) oil. This will increase your intake of the omega-3 fatty acids which the body cannot make and which is one of the more difficult nutrients to source from the diet. You can take it in liquid or capsule form, and should aim for the equivalent of 1,000mg, three times a day.

Herbs are often best taken in liquid tincture form, which is the fastest route into the bloodstream. Take 30 drops of Ginkgo biloba, three times a day, as well as 20 drops of the prostate-protecting herb, Saw palmetto, also three times a day. Also investigate a herb called Damiana, which can help increase sensitivity.

The antioxidant vitamin E also plays an important role in male sexual health. Sufferers should take the equivalent of 500iu a day, with the main meal. Bloating and stomach problems may be a sign of over-fermentation in the body, which can also interfere with sexual performance. If a man complains of a 'heavy feeling', especially after eating, he needs to avoid yeast-rich beer and bread for a while and monitor any improvements. Following all these measures for three months should produce a dramatic improvement.

Fasting DeTox Diet

This is a DeTox diet for those who consider themselves well but who would benefit from a holistic spring-clean. Devised specifically for me by David Crawford, the UK-based nutritionist and a pioneer of True Nutrition – that is using natural foods, not supplements for health – it is an excellent introduction to the idea of fasting which is the ideal way to rid the body of toxins, fast. I must stress, though, that if you are not in good health or have not fasted before, *do not* embark on this programme without the supervision of a medical practitioner or your holistic health therapist. If, however, you have detoxed before, and relish the prospect of a gentle but effective spring-clean, here goes.

Choose which week you plan to DeTox and mark it in your diary. This particular programme works well at the end of March and in early April, when you can include the beneficial properties of fresh, young herbs and shoots such as parsley, sage, sorrel, lamb's lettuce and even nettle in your salads. This is the time of year when all these plants are bursting with energy-giving nutrients.

Getting Started

Early Morning For the two days before your DeTox begins, start your day with the juice of half an organic lemon dissolved in a small glass of warm water. Half an hour later, juice equal parts of carrots and apples, making enough to fill a half-pint glass. (Always juice your own fruits. Do not rely on ready-made, shop-bought products.)

Mid-morning Snack from a selection of unsulphured dried fruits, which you need to have soaked overnight in tepid water. You are also going to make a nutritious, detoxing drink by blending ground almond nuts (also pre-soaked for 24 hours) and coconut milk. Add the latter to suit your own taste.

In these initial, preparatory stages you can eat lunch as usual if you want to. It is probably better though, to skip it altogether and confine yourself to fresh fruit if you feel hungry again in the afternoon. You can eat any fruit of your choice but, for this particular detox, avoid citrus fruits, which have been shown to be the cause of hidden food intolerances in many people, particularly those prone to digestive disorders. Your evening meal should be as usual, but avoid animal meats and animal by-products.

Bedtime About half an hour before bedtime, prepare an equal-parts combination of carrot and celery juice to make about half a pint. Again, juice your own fruit.

At no time during this two-day preparation should you have caffeine in any form, refined sugar, artificial sweeteners, alcohol or any other form of stimulating beverage. Herbal teas are OK, and you need to try and drink a minimum of 1.5 litres of still, filtered water. (You will be trying to maintain this level of fluids throughout the detox plan.)

Days 1, 2 & 3

Start your day with half a pint of warm water and then begin your fast, eating no food and drinking only water for each of the first three days. If you are new to fasting, this will play havoc with your taste buds but you will be pleasantly surprised to discover you are not suffering from hunger pangs at all.

Day 4

You are now ready to return to part of the preparatory regimen, starting your day with the warm water and lemon. Allow a break of 30 minutes and then juice equal parts of carrots and apples. Pre-soak more unsulphured dried fruits and make the same almond nut and coconut milk blended drink for your mid-morning nourishment if you wish. Otherwise, eat nothing until lunchtime.

Lunch It is important to take the time and trouble to prepare this critical first post-fasting lunch in advance.

Preparation:
- pre-soak a quarter cup of sprouted sesame seeds for 12 hours
- pre-soak half a cup of sprouted chickpeas for 24 hours
- pre-soak a quarter cup of celery seeds for 12 hours
- pre-soak a quarter cup of fenugreek seeds for 24 hours
- pre-soak half a cup of mung beans for 24 hours

Rinse all the above thoroughly to wash off any traces of tannins that may linger in some of the seed casings. Mix them in a large bowl and add grated raw carrot, beetroot and cabbage. Toss with some fresh lamb's lettuce salad leaves and other fresh, young herbs to your own taste. Add a small amount of cold-pressed virgin olive oil if desired. Because you have fasted for three days, you may find this salad too filling. Only eat what you can comfortably manage.

Do not eat again in the afternoon following this lunch, but keep up your intake of pure water. In the evening, eat fresh fruit and wait for an hour before eating some pre-soaked almonds and a little of the left-over lunchtime salad. End your day with the carrot and celery juice you first made in the preparatory period before the fast.

Day 5

Start and end your day with the same juices as for Day 4. You may find you now want to interchange your morning dried fruit and blended coconut milk drink with lunch, omitting one of them. This is perfectly acceptable. You may not be eating much compared with your normal intake but it will seem very filling because of your long fast. If you have decided to skip your lunchtime salad, prepare a raw hummus to eat with fresh salad shoots and some sticks of celery in the evening.

Supper Once again, you need to prepare the raw hummus in advance of your mealtime.

- 1 cup of pre-soaked (24 hours) chickpeas
- half a cup of pre-soaked (12 hours) sesame seeds. You can, if you prefer, use organic tahini
- half a teaspoon of fresh lemon juice

Blend the chickpeas and sesame seeds (or tahini) into a creamy paste. You decide on the consistency that appeals to you. Finally, add the lemon juice and blend for another 30 seconds.

If you have opted for dried fruit only at lunchtime, then you must have a salad in the evening.

Day 6

Try and fast again. If this it too taxing, keep to the same regimen, reducing the amount of salads, nuts and fruit you are eating but sticking to the exact same quantities of juices.

Day 7

On the last day of your week-long DeTox, you revert back to the eating patterns of the 4th and 5th days, eating as much or as little as you wish of these combinations of foods. Again, do not vary the quantities of the morning and bedtime juices.

To End

The idea is to ease back into your normal eating programme by keeping as much of the energy-giving and detoxifying foods from the previous week in your diet as you can face. Try even harder to keep the juicing going and make sure you are drinking 1.5 litres of water (in winter) and at least 2 litres in summer. It is also an excellent idea to incorporate one day of fasting every week in your normal life. Choose your special day and stick to it. It can take several weeks for your body to adjust to the new routine, but it will adapt and accept that for one day a week, the only thing it can expect is pure water.

The reason you eat so much fruit in this detox is that fruits help to cleanse the system. They have a high carbon content that 'burns off' lingering debris in the body. They should really only be eaten when ripe. Vegetables are the body-building foods. They have higher proportions of protein-building materials and less carbon than fruit.

If you are worried about fasting for the first time, do get professional advice. (For tailor-made fasting and detox programmes, consult a qualified nutritionist.) However, the body has its own neat biochemical mechanism for making sure you are not going to expire with hunger. To help during times of fasting, the body makes a compound called ketone which automatically suppresses the appetite. Ketones are the broken-down products of fatty acids. When you fast, the body releases more of these substances into the bloodstream, which stops you from suffering the misery of hunger pangs. If you do not feel comfortable with a three-day fast, try just one day and adapt this plan to suit your own needs.

Fertility

Nutritionists frequently tell me that women who come to them to tackle some other disorder – say a problem with their skin or digestion – end up pregnant just a few months after changing their eating habits. I wonder then, how the live baby 'hit' rate of the nutrition centres compares with the more expensive private fertility clinics.

The problem, according to Dr Gillian McKeith, a US-trained nutritionist and author of *10 Steps to Perfect Health for New Moms* is often linked to a major vitamin or mineral deficiency or an overload of toxic metals such as mercury or lead (see page 88), which can interfere with the conception process.

'People have no idea how easy it is to get pregnant as long as there are no medical blocks,' she says, which is reassuring for those diagnosed with unexplained infertility. She continues:

'The usual problem in conceiving is that they just don't eat properly. I have women who come along complaining of bloating, excessive gas and tiredness, and when you do the biochemical work what you find is that they are hugely deficient in minerals, vitamins and health-promoting bacteria in the gut.

'They come for one problem and we then discover that fertility is a problem too, until we start to use nutrition, herbs and the right kind of food combining to redress these imbalances. The men come along describing watery, non-viable semen – which again we can correct as long as both parties are willing to make the necessary dietary and lifestyle changes.'

In about 40% of cases, the male partner is reckoned to be grossly deficient in the nutrients which nourish healthy sperm, especially zinc which affects every aspect of reproductive health, including the longevity of sperm in the vaginal tract. It is lost during ejaculation and also has a kind of domino effect in the body so that levels of other minerals, especially magnesium (which influences how sperm clumps together) will also be low, verging on deficient. In both partners, the main problem may be one of malabsorption. The important thing, says McKeith, is to get the body back to optimum health so it can absorb the nutrients you do eat, and to then keep it free of toxins.

When, for example, Foresight – the UK's Association for the Promotion of Preconceptual Care, which boasts a 90% success rate with couples having trouble conceiving – conducted a survey of couples asking for help, it found that nine out of every 15 men contacting the group were suffering some form of genito-urinary infection. What the Association euphemistically refers to as 'Grubby Lifestyles' includes obvious toxins such as alcohol, tobacco and cannabis, but also infections with names that sound more like flowers but which, if left unchecked, can lead to permanent infertility.

These include the sexually-transmitted *chlamydia*, which can cause scarring and blockage of the Fallopian tubes in women, increasing the risk of an ectopic pregnancy, and *gardnerella*, which has been implicated in causing infertility by preventing the implantation of the embryo in the thickened lining of the uterus.

Dr Marilyn Glenville, current chairman of Foresight and a nutritional therapist specialising in women's hormonal health and infertility, advises that both parties should be screened for these types of infection before even trying to conceive, particularly if there is a history of miscarriage.

As well as zinc, she says that when fertility is a problem, both sexes are also frequently deficient in the potent antioxidant selenium, which can be found in brazil nuts, pumpkin seeds, kidneys and liver, and which is now the subject of a major Cancer Research Campaign-sponsored UK trial investigating its efficacy in fighting cancer.

She recommends both sexes supplement their diet with at least 100mcg of selenium and 15mg of zinc, which can help regulate hormonal imbalances in women and which is so crucial for sperm health in men. She says – and I agree

– that even one alcoholic drink a week is one too many if you are trying to conceive, and suggests couples give themselves four months to improve their health before trying to get pregnant.

This is one area where conventional and complementary treatments really can work together. I think people who have been told they are suffering from unexplained infertility get rushed into IVF or into taking ovulation-boosting drugs, when what they should be doing, is going right back to the foundation of their health and looking at what they eat, what they drink, their jobs which may bring them into contact with harmful chemicals, and their lifestyles, which may be doing the same.

Sperm counts have slumped by almost 50% in the last five decades, and even when no problems have been detected it now takes the average seemingly healthy couple 11-12 months to conceive. According to Dr Glenville, vitamin E supplements have been shown to help fertilization. In one study by researchers at the University of Sheffield, it was found that taking high doses of vitamin E – 600mg every day for three months – improved the quality of sperm in 20% of men with poor sperm performance.

One theory for the dramatic decline in sperm health is that xeno-oestrogens are to blame. These are toxins produced by chemicals used in the environment and in food processing and packaging which have an oestrogenic-like effect on the body. Men are advised to minimise their contact with these chemicals by switching to an organic diet and by avoiding foods stored in plastic containers.

Amino acids are the building blocks of protein in the body. Those which have been identified as being crucial to healthy sperm include L-arginine and L-taurine. You can take supplements of both, but natural sources of L-arginine include chocolate, brown rice, oatmeal, raisins, sunflower and sesame seeds, while eggs, organic meats (especially pork and lamb) shellfish and organic milk are all high in L-taurine.

Living foods are an excellent nutritional boost to reproductive health in both sexes, according to Dr McKeith, who has formulated a Living Food Energy Powder that she gives to all prospective mums. Derived from the kind of nourishing foods few of us make an effort to eat – including live, sprouted foods such as millet, quinoa, flax, seaweeds and algae – and then formulated with essential nutrients such as zinc, vitamin E, calcium, magnesium and iron, patients who have trouble conceiving are advised to take three teaspoonfuls a day. You will also need to cut out coffee (just two cups a day has been shown to reduce fertility by 50%), alcohol and mucus-forming dairy foods.

Red clover, which has a high vitamin content, can help re-establish fertility and will balance the acid/alkaline levels of the vagina and uterus. High in protein, calcium and magnesium, it also provides these important nutrients in a form which is easily absorbable. If you are not ovulating, the herb Agnus castus is a potent regulator of hormones.

Fibroids

Most people think of these particular tumours as forming only in the womb, but in fact they are actually abnormal muscle cells and can form anywhere in the pelvic cavity. In 50% of sufferers there are no symptoms. In the remainder, severe PMT, low blood-sugar levels, heavy, painful periods, painful sexual intercourse and bleeding between periods are all common. So, too, are anaemia, fatigue and fertility problems. Experts are at a loss to explain why the condition is five times more common in women of African origin, but most now agree there could be a powerful genetic factor at work.

In most cases, fibroids appear in the late 30s and 40s and then shrink after menopause. So why are surgeons so quick to whip out the womb? (In the US, 30% of all hysterectomies are for the removal of fibroids.) Sufferers need to resist a knee-jerk reaction, and, instead, first try a diet that supports hormone balance with little or no animal fats and only high-quality, unpolluted fish oils. The liver will probably need supporting, too, so take 200mg of the herb milk thistle twice a day.

A combination of the amino acid L-arginine (500mg on an empty stomach) together with 50mg of vitamin B_6 daily and up to 5g of vitamin C will also enhance immune function and retard the growth of existing fibroids. Vitamin A (25,000 iu) is also used to restore the body's connective tissue to normal functioning.

Do not take L-arginine if you suffer from cold sores. It can activate the herpes simplex virus. High doses of vitamin C can cause stomach upsets.

Fungal Infections

Repeated fungal infections can be a sign of diabetes, so check with your physician to rule this out as the underlying cause. The medical name for a fungal infection is *Mycosis* and if you've ever had one, you will know how hard they are to eradicate.

A treatment using a supplement called Molkosan, which contains a concentrated form of fungus-fighting whey, can be very effective, restoring the skin to a clear condition within a few short weeks.

One of the most common fungal infections is, of course, athlete's foot. To treat with Molkosan, soak absorbent cotton in the liquid of the whey supplement, bind it to the affected part and leave on overnight. Alternate treating the affected areas with Molkosan and Echinacea. According to many naturopathic doctors there is no quicker solution for many persistent fungal problems. The same holds true for other skin blemishes and infections.

Gout

Gout was always thought of as a disease of affluence – a sign you had over indulged by eating and drinking too much. In fact, it is a form of arthritis caused by an excess of uric acid, which is itself a byproduct of a substance called purine which is found in certain foods, including meat, asparagus, anchovies, chicken and mushrooms.

A fault in the way uric acid is broken down causes both uric acid and *urates* (uric acid salts) to accumulate in the bloodstream and the joints. This slowly destroys the joints and causes deposits of salt in the skin and the cartilage, especially in the big toe. The number of cases of gout has doubled in the West over the last 30 years. For some people, even a small amount of the wrong food can trigger an attack.

Prescription drugs are used either to increase the excretion of uric acid or slow down the rate at which urates form, but you can also use supplements and foods to help prevent further flare-ups. Cherry juice, for example, lowers uric acid levels. Celery juice, which promotes the flow of urine through the kidneys, can also relieve symptoms. Buying a good juicer will help increase your dietary intake of both these foods.

Avoiding the wrong foods, particularly those high in purine, can help. These include legumes, liver, mackerel, sardines, shrimp, sweetbreads, asparagus, bran, cauliflower, saltwater fish, meat, spinach and whole grains. Eat less protein and drink more fluids to help flush excess uric acid from your body. Carrying too much weight will also exacerbate the problem, so keep yours under control.

Hair Dyes

During research for my honours degree, I carried out laboratory-controlled tests on commercial hair dyes which we were investigating for carcinogenic activity. We found that even weak solutions caused mutations in the bacteria we were monitoring. Ever since then, I have had concerns about chemical hair colouring.

Of course, these were not published or peer-reviewed results, but they were enough for me to wonder if I was the only user of hair dyes who might be concerned. Of course I was not, and with good reason. According to Samuel Epstein and David Steinmann, authors of *The Safe Shopper's Bible*, a lifetime's use of permanent and semi-permanent hair dyes, particularly dark and black colours, has been linked with an increased risk of cancer, especially non-Hodgkin's lymphoma, multiple myeloma, leukaemia and Hodgkin's disease. There is also evidence of an increased risk of breast cancer.

Temporary dyes and rinses contain chemicals such as Acid Orange 87, Solvent Brown 44, Avid Blue 168 and Acid Violet 73, which have all shown carcinogenic activity and which should be avoided. Bleaches are safer than dyes, with few if any long-term risks, and hair colourings using pure henna, camomile and other herbs are safe. Also, women who start to dye their hair in their 20s have more than twice the risk of developing an associated cancer than those who delay until their 40s.

You could revert to one of the natural henna dyes – although even henna is not always what it seems. Black henna, for example, is not henna at all but is made from the leaves of another plant called senna, which is also used as a laxative. Variations on the distinctive and tell-tale henna red, which not everyone wants to sport, will have been adulterated with other dyes. Thankfully, there are a number of manufacturers now recognising that women want to cover grey hair or simply change their hair colour without taking this risk. A list of those supplying dyes deemed to be safest of all can be found in the Resources chapter.

Hair Loss

Hair loss may be caused by an underactive thyroid gland. The thyroid hormones are made from, among other things, iodine and the amino acid, tyrosine. These hormones regulate metabolism in every single cell. Your doctor can do a simple basal body temperature test to find out if this is your problem. If it is, supplements of a sea vegetable called kelp can help since, like most seaweeds, it is a very rich natural source of iodine. It also contains potassium, magnesium, calcium and iron. Take according to the directions on the bottle.

You might also want to pay a visit to your fishmonger, because other natural sources of iodine include clams, lobsters, oysters and sardines. Regular exercise will also stimulate thyroid gland secretions and increase the sensitivity of your body's tissues, including your hair follicles, to the thyroid hormones.

It makes sense to put more of an emphasis on scalp care. Sufferers need to adopt a more holistic approach by investigating the underlying cause of hair loss – which is often dietary – before spending a fortune on creams and shampoos.

The UK tricologist David Satchell claims a 70% success rate (the highest in the world) for the treatment of alopecia. The key to the treatment programme he has devised at his Eucaderm clinic is alternating hot and cold water head massages. They sound awful, of course, but they really do work by stimulating increased blood flow to the hair follicles in the scalp. According to Satchell, you should dunk your head for 10 to 15 seconds in hot and then cold water, five times per session. To counter scalp problems, including hair loss, aim for as many sessions in a day as you can manage. Otherwise, for general maintenance, do this just once a day and avoid using detergent shampoos.

You need to get more live enzymes into your diet by stepping up the amount of raw fruit and vegetables you eat. You can also achieve this through juicing and by taking a good multisupplement that comes with live enzymes.

Hangover Cures

Alcohol is a diuretic, which means it forces fluids out of the body. When this happens, you lose lots of potassium which you need to keep the body fluids balanced. Bananas are an excellent source of this mineral (just one will provide half the recommended daily dose), and a Traditional Chinese remedy for hangovers is to boil them in their skins to make a tea from the liquid. Bananas also replenish lost magnesium, which helps control blood sugar levels that are wiped out by booze. Vitamin C will make you feel better too; again, bananas are a good source. The flesh is sweet and will help rebalance the body's blood sugar levels, which have been decimated by your night on the tiles.

What Really Works When It's Really Bad?

Prairie Oyster with a Hint of Hair of the Dog!

1 shot of olive oil
1-2 tablespoons of tomato ketchup
1 raw egg yolk (don't break this)
salt, pepper

tabasco

worcestershire sauce

vinegar or lemon juice

The olive oil acts as a liver and gallbladder flush. (It's so effective, it can even trigger the expulsion and excretion of gallbladder stones!) The raw egg contains an amino acid called N-acetyl-cysteine (NAC). This is one of the building-blocks of a natural compound called glutathione. In the body this acts as a major mine-sweeper, clearing out toxins from alcohol and cigarette smoke. Ironically, when you drink you lower levels of this nutrient, so building it up again is a good idea, especially since a much-quoted study into hangover cures by *New Scientist* magazine showed NAC was the best antidote of all. The tomato ketchup provides bioflavanoids or vitamin P. These are superb antioxidants in their own right, which means they boost the immune system and again, clear out those damaging toxins. If you can't get going without the hair of the dog, add a splash of vodka, which contains fewer congeners (or additives) than any other alcoholic drink. This explains why you get less of a hangover if you stick to this spirit. If you're in a rush and don't have time to mix a Prairie Oyster, boiling vinegar and inhaling the steam will at least get rid of that hangover headache.

Not everyone can face the prospect of a raw egg, which can contain other health hazards anyway. Fortunately, the supplement-makers have come up with a tablet solution: a product called Intox RX. This also provides the liver-protecting herb, milk thistle, which has been shown in trials to regenerate damaged liver cells.

Extreme Measures – The Upward Purge

Rich and fashionable Romans who were famed for their bacchanalian feasts built themselves special rooms in which to indulge in the 'upward purge'. These rooms, known as vomitories, always had a marble rail over which my lord or lady could drape themselves while a slave tickled the back of their throat. After drinking a few soothing glasses of warm water to recover from the effort of what is called an emetic, they would return to their partying.

A high enema (use your imagination) achieved much the same results, but the herbal emetic is less gross. I suggest (if you decide this is the only solution for you) that you use mustard, which should do the job in no time at all. You need to drink four or five glasses of mustard juice until you retch. If you can't stomach the idea of mustard, salt might just do the trick. If this fails – and you don't have a Roman slave to hand – try the finger at the back of the throat.

Once you've had your upward purge and cleansed your system, you'll need to soothe yourself with a gentle cup of peppermint tea (this is antispasmodic and will settle your stomach again). A few drops of a herb called Goldenseal, dissolved in juice or water, will then destroy the mucus and fermentation in the stomach which, if left unchecked, will irritate the gut and make you feel nauseated. Once done, you can get back to the big party or go to bed without feeling sick.

Before You Party

Take steps to reduce your hangover *before* you go out by taking a natural remedy called Kudzu. Used by Chinese healers to suppress alcohol cravings, it contains two phytochemicals, daidzin and daidzen, which will eliminate the worst symptoms, including the nausea, headache and sickness. Artichoke can also soothe a gut that has been irritated by alcohol. In new clinical studies, the active ingredient (cynarin) was shown to increase bile production into the duodenum of healthy volunteers. Researchers suggest this could be a useful treatment for many other dyspeptic conditions, including irritable colon and flatulence.

Simple Standbys

Boiled rabbit droppings and pickled sheep's eyes are among the more bizarre medieval hangover cures. Here are some less stomach-churning quick fixes if you've been daft enough to get drunk:

a sugar cube soaked in painkilling and mind-numbing clove oil, which you suck on

lavender honey – take a teaspoon every half hour, through the night. The honey will keep blood sugar levels up; lavender is an excellent all-round healing herb and responds to the body's needs at any particular time. It can, for example, ease nausea, headaches and indigestion, and works to counter the depressive activity of alcohol.

gentian bitters can quell nausea, while dandelion tincture, which is a
rich source of potassium, will help re-regulate the body's fluids.

dandelion leaves – rich source of minerals, especially potassium to
re-regulate fluids. Make a tea or eat salad made from young leaves.

fresh sprig of parsley – chew on this to freshen the breath and soothe
the digestion.

If you really need to sober up fast, make a tea from the fresh or dried
organic peel of a grapefruit. It is loaded with vitamin C and also
contains phenolics which help the body produce its own detoxifying
compounds.

Immunity Boosting

A weakened immune system leaves the body vulnerable to virtually every type of
illness and disease, especially when you move between climates, countries and
time zones. Even the shift from late summer to autumn is always marked in the
health calendar by the arrival of a new generation of viruses causing coughs
and colds.

Although the immune system can recognise viral strains it has encountered and
beaten off before, it will not recognise a virus which has mutated and even the
smallest genetic change will trick the immune system into thinking a brand new

species, for which it has no antibodies, has landed. While a strong immune system will cope with this attack, one that has been weakened by poor nutrition and too much stress will struggle to get you back to good health.

Fatigue, lethargy, repeated infections, slow wound-healing, allergies, thrush, colds and flu are all signs that the body's immune system is functioning below par. A healthy adult, for example, should suffer no more than two colds a year, so if you do succumb to every passing infection, you definitely need to start supporting your immune system.

Almost everyone has now heard of the best-selling herbal remedy, echinacea, which in Germany is prescribed by doctors and pharmacists to help fight colds and flu. It is effective, as long as you don't overuse it, but I find another less glamorous herb even more so. Goldenseal, which was once used to treat syphillis and gonorrhoea, was first discovered by Aboriginal healers in Australia. It will not only help prevent an infection if you are feeling low, but can reduce the inflammation of mucus membranes once you have a cough or cold.

Most people will also reach for the vitamin C tablets at the first sign of a splutter. A quarter of a century ago, the US Nobel Laureate Linus Pauling caused an outcry among medics by claiming that this nutrient, taken in high enough doses, could alleviate the symptoms of the common cold. This debate continues, but what we do now know is that many of the symptoms of a cold have nothing to do with the cold virus itself, but are caused by the body's own immune response to that alien invader. It is this secondary problem that vitamin C can help counter.

What happens is that during a cold the mucus membranes which line the nose become charged with the white blood cells that release large amounts of chemicals designed to destroy the virus. Unfortunately, these substances also attack the cells of the mucus membranes themselves, causing a runny nose and other disturbances. So the idea behind giving antioxidants such as vitamins C, A and E to tackle a cold is two-fold. First, these nutrients have now been shown to support the immune system. Just as importantly, they weaken the body's immune attack on its own tissues.

Poor nutrition is the most common cause of a weakened immune reponse. Foods that are good natural sources of the immune-boosting antioxidants include kiwi fruits (which contain more vitamin C than oranges), Chinese cabbage (an excellent source of vitamin A) and avocado, known as nature's own superfood because it provides the optimum healthy ratio of fat, carbohydrate, protein and vitamin E. Foods that are rich in vitamin B_6, which boosts the production of antibodies to fight infection, will also help. These foods include bananas, carrots, lentils, tuna, salmon, wholegrain flour and sunflower seeds. You also need to step up your intake of dietary zinc by eating more seafood, eggs, turkey, pumpkin seeds and crabmeat.

How to Beat A Cold and Boost Immunity

Goldenseal It tastes vile and will stain your fingers bright yellow, but Goldenseal is highly effective. Take it in liquid or capsule form. If you prefer liquid, you can buy a wild-crafted Goldenseal (this simply means it is harvested naturally from the wild, not cultivated, which herbalists believe gives it even greater potency). Do not, though, self-dose with this herb if you are pregnant or have high blood pressure.

Antioxidants The body cannot store vitamin C for longer than three weeks but must rely on your dietary intake. To prevent winter infections, take 1,000mg a day. To boost the immune system and ward off colds, you'll find it hard to beat a product called Well-max by Country Life (see Resources), which combines all the antioxidants plus antibacterial grapeseed extract, Goldenseal, Siberian ginseng, astralagus, schizandra, Shi'take and Reishi mushrooms, plus bee propolis, garlic, echinacea and the liver-supporting herb, pau d'arco.

Echinacea Also known as purple coneflower, echinacea is the top-selling herb in the US. Introduced into medical practice in 1887, modern research into how it supports the immune system began in the 1930s in Germany – where, by the mid-1990s for example, it was being prescribed by doctors and pharmacists 2.5 million times to fight colds and flu. Said to work by increasing the numbers and the activity of white blood cells, it also increases the production of interferon, a chemical which is critical to the immune system response. At the onset of a cold, take 20 drops of echinacea tincture, 3–4 times a day for 10–14 days. To prevent a cold, take 3 times a day for 6 to 8 weeks – but make sure you have 'rest' periods or the protective effects will diminish.

Maitake One of the more exotic immune-boosting supplements to get noticed in the West is the Maitake mushroom (*Grifoloa frondosa*) which grows to the size of a basketball, deep in the mountains of northeastern Japan. Highly prized for its immune-boosting properties, it has been shown to stimulate the immune response by activating the T-cells – the body's own defence against viruses and cancer cells. Recent animal studies reveal that combining maitake extract with chemotherapy treatment resulted in a 99% tumour shrinkage in just 14 days. Studies in the US, Japan and the UK have also shown that giving maitake extract to HIV patients can help protect the body's disease-fighting T-cells, which the HIV virus normally destroys. Said to improve liver function, too, it contains powerful polysaccharides (chemicals known to boost the immune system) and is currently in clinical trials with both HIV and cancer patients. The recommended dosage is between 3–7g per day.

Cat's Claw A herb which grows in the rain forests of South America, the active constituents are the oxyindole alkaloids which stimulate immune function. Not to be taken by pregnant or lactating women, it has both anti-inflammatory and anti-oxidant properties, making it useful for wound-healing. To make a therapeutic tea, boil 1g of cat's claw root bark with 250ml (1 cup) of water for 15 minutes. Cool, strain and drink. Take three cups a day. Alternatively, take 1–2ml of tincture twice a day, or 20–60mg of standardised extract daily.

Aloe Vera A veritable storehouse of vitamins, minerals, amino acids, enzymes and numerous other ingredients, aloe vera acts as both an immune-enhancer and a natural antiseptic. Recommended for serious immune-deficiency conditions, including Chronic Fatigue Syndrome, drink a quarter of a glass each morning and increase the dosage by drinking the same amount again at the end of the day if you feel a cold or other infection threatening. Find a product that is high in the mucopolysaccharides which bolster the body's natural defences.

Grapefruit Seed Extract (Citricidal) An antibiotic, antiviral and antifungal agent recommended for stomach bugs, throat and ear infections, and cold sores; you should only take this when you feel ill. If travelling to any country where you are worried about food hygiene, take 75mg three times a day for a month before you go and continue for another month after your return. The active ingredients are called Proanthocyanidins, a class of nutrients which belong to the flavanoid family and whose primary function is to work as antioxidants in the body, mopping up the free radical toxic byproducts of metabolism. Available in tablet – or better still, liquid – form. Take 15 drops in a glass of water, 2–3 times a day.

L-Arginine An amino acid which promotes wound-healing and which supports the immune system. Dairy, meat, poultry and fish are all good natural sources. Levels drop during times of increased stress, making supplementation important. It works by stimulating the thymus gland, which in turn stores the disease-fighting T-lymphocytes until they are needed to fight infection. Also used to treat sexual dysfunction and infertility in men, the recommended dose is 3–6g a day.

Warning: Some researchers believe that L-arginine can trigger a herpes infection so avoid if you already suffer from cold sores.

Probiotics Beneficial bacteria which help boost immune function are called probiotics. They alter the balance of microflora in the gut by inhibiting the growth of harmful bacteria and favouring those which, instead, aid digestion and promote a healthy immune response to infection. Frequently used to repopulate the digestive tract after a course of antibiotics has upset this balance, research has shown they can prevent up to 50% of the infections that are common after antibiotic use. They can also be used by travellers to avoid diarrhoea. Found naturally in fermented foods, yoghurt is a traditional source – although many products contain no live bacteria at all. Even those products claiming to provide millions of live bacteria may not work since these can be destroyed by the acid in the stomach. Seven Seas, better known for its fish oils, has now developed a capsule with an enteric coating which protects the bacteria through the stomach so they reach the place they are needed – the colon. If you prefer to take a powder, take 8g per day of recognised strain such as *Lactobacillus acidophilus*.

Liquorice   Particularly effective when the immune system is suppressed by stress or steroids, this herb has been shown to have an antibiotic effect against throat infections, candida and herpes simplex (the virus which causes cold sores when your immune system is run down). It can relieve a dry, irritating cough and is also a good lung tonic. Only take it when you feel ill; chew one 200-300mg tablet, three times a day, before meals.

Glutamine   Critical for both normal brain and immune function, this nutrient is amazingly versatile. It is also a component of glutathione, the body's primary antioxidant, present in virtually every single cell. It is often given to burns patients to promote wound-healing and is now available in a powerful immune-boosting combination with anthocyanidins. These are found naturally in red/blue foods such as red grapes, beetroot and berries, which are also very good for the lungs. Anthocyanidins also remove the free radical scavenger molecules which would otherwise pollute the body and lower its natural resistance to disease.

Herbal Teas   You can easily make your own immune-boosting herbal teas. Try ginger and cinnamon tea, which you make by putting four large slices of ginger and a small stick of cinnamon into boiling water. Allow to 'brew' for 15 minutes. Cat's Claw tea from the *Uncaria tomentosa* plant is another powerful immune system stimulant; drink it sweetened with apple or blackcurrant concentrate.

Kombucha Tea   The Kombucha or Manchurian 'mushroom' is now used by millions of people to boost immunity. The name is misleading: it is not a mushroom at all but a large, flat, pancake-shaped fungus-like growth that is a combination of health-promoting lichen, beneficial bacteria and yeast. Used in Asia as a natural energy booster, it is brewed into a strong antiviral and antibacterial tea after it has been left to ferment for a week or so in a mixture of water, sugar, apple cider vinegar and green or black tea. Now also widely used in the West to help fight immune-related diseases such as Chronic Fatigue and Multiple Sclerosis (MS), some devotees claim it can even help reverse the ageing process. Kombucha Tea Networks – they exist in the UK, Australia, South Africa and the US – can get you started with a handbook and starter culture. For more details see Resources.

Insomnia

Every night, millions of people go to bed knowing they will spend the next eight hours tossing and turning and wondering when they will ever get another good night's sleep. Insomnia is one of the more common everyday problems and is estimated to affect one in every three adults at some point in their lives. Researchers have now identified some 80 different sleep disorders including chronic insomnia, which is believed to affect 15% of the adult population.

The condition is said to be chronic if it continues for longer than three weeks. If you cannot sleep for just a few nights, your insomnia is said to be transient; if you cannot sleep for a week or two, it is deemed a short-term problem. The latter two types of insomnia are almost always prompted by an outside event. Worrying about giving a presentation at work, for example, may cost you one or two nights' sleep. The death of a parent may disrupt your sleep patterns for a few weeks.

The underlying causes of chronic insomnia are more difficult to pinpoint and tackle, but they can include depression, a dietary overload of stimulants, especially caffeine, drinking too much alcohol, chronic pain due to other causes, muscle cramps and other physical ailments. Researchers, though, suggest that at least 50% of all cases of chronic insomnia are caused by psychological factors, especially depression and anxiety.

The body's circadian rhythm (which determines when you sleep and when you wake) is controlled by a hormone called melatonin, which is, in turn, released by the pea-sized pineal gland which lies at the top of the brain. As with other hormones, levels of melatonin decrease with age. By the age of 60, for example, your body produces half the amount of melatonin it did when you were 20. It has been shown that tiny doses – just 0.3mg – of replacement melatonin taken at bedtime can quickly bring blood levels of the hormone back to normal and help induce a good night's sleep. Patients taking melatonin in supplement form report they have less trouble getting to sleep in the first place – they drop off in less than half the time it takes without it – they sleep longer and they wake up feeling more alert and refreshed.

Lots of long-haul travellers use melatonin to re-regulate their body clocks and avoid the worst disorientations of jet-lag, and the supplement is perfect for shift-workers and businessmen and -women who regularly travel long-haul for short periods of time and have to be alert enough to shift into a new time zone and attend meetings. Its short-term use, for up to a week, has been deemed safe and without side-effects, but if you live in the UK where over-the-counter sales of melatonin are illegal, it is only available by private prescription.

You get round this problem by taking a step back in the biochemistry of the brain and, instead of boosting levels of melatonin with a melatonin supplement, you increase levels by stepping up your intake of *serotonin*, a neurotransmitter involved in the manufacture of melatonin. You can also use diet to boost levels of tryptophan, an amino-acid which is itself critical for the manufacture of serotonin.

Researchers have found, for example, that people who find it hard to get off to sleep are usually deficient in their levels of serotonin, the synthesis of which also requires large amounts of vitamin B_6 (pyridoxine) which is found in carrots, cheese, avocado, fish, lentils, peas, potatoes, spinach, sunflower seeds and wholemeal flour. If you suffer from insomnia, eat more of these foods and cut out the high-sugar foods such as white bread and white rice, which can cause fluctuations in blood-sugar levels. Stick instead to a high-carbohydrate diet to maximise the presence of L-tryptophan, a form of tryptophan used in the brain. In fact, those who eat a carbohydrate-based diet of quality wholefoods are found to be calmer, rarely depressed and better able to sleep soundly than those who do not.

Turkey meat contains a large amount of tryptophan, which might explain why adult members of the family fall asleep straight after the traditional Christmas or Thanksgiving meal. Combining it with complex carbohydrate, say a spoonful of honey, will enhance the effect by increasing blood sugar levels, which, in turn, causes the pancreas to release more insulin. This then has the knock-on effect of chasing several of the amino acids that would normally compete with tryptophan for receptor sites in the brain from the blood into the liver, leaving the coast clear for tryptophan to dominate. This is one of the finest examples of psychonutrition – using food to influence mood – that I can think of.

Most of us only get a third of the optimum daily dose of calcium our bodies need, and calcium deficiency has long been linked with increased tension and sleep disturbances. Calcium is a potent sleep-inducer – this explains why drinking a glass of warmed milk at bedtime can help – and should be taken as calcium citrate or calcium hydroxyapatite (two of the forms the body can most easily absorb). In Russia, the folk remedy is to grind anise and serve it with warm milk and honey. Milk is not only high in calcium but rich in tryptophan, and so has a doubly powerful tranquillising effect.

The list of herbal remedies which can help promote a good night's sleep is impressive and ranges from everyday offerings such as mint, rosemary and the antispasmodic muscle-relaxant thyme to the more exotic passionflower (for chronic insomnia) and saffron. Camomile, once planted on graves in ancient England as a symbol that the deceased would be reborn, is an excellent natural sedative and safe to give to children. You can make a tea from the flowers or, for super-potency, juice the herb in the same way you would juice wheat grass to make a nutritional drink. Fresh lemon balm is also an excellent remedy.

In the East, a hot foot bath is a traditional remedy for insomnia – the logic is that it draws the chi or energy from the brain to calm a racing mind – and if you enjoy using essential oils when bathing, both lavender and lemon balm will help relax you. If you prefer a homoeopathic remedy, Lycopodium is the one most frequently prescribed for anyone who spends half the night going over the previous day, drops off in the small hours of the morning only to wake and start worrying again at around 4a.m.

Sleeplessness is a natural feature of ageing. The majority of sleeping pills are prescribed to the over-65s, who may find that a late-night snack will help.

Researchers at the Massachusetts Institute of Technology (MIT) in Cambridge, Boston, have shown that an English muffin or a banana before bedtime, for example, can greatly improve the quality of sleep.

Too much stress produces too much adrenaline in the body, high levels of which overpower the serotonin that would normally help you get a good night's sleep. Bringing your stress levels under control is therefore important. The technique that has proved the most effective in regulating the disturbed sleep patterns of airline pilots is a technique called Autogenic Training (see Resources).

Certain prescription drugs, including oral contraceptives and beta-blockers, may play havoc with sleep patterns. Caffeine, which stimulates the production of more adrenaline, is a major culprit in the sleep wars. If you are drinking around 12 cups a day, you are ingesting a gram of caffeine, which is more than enough to keep you awake and counting sheep. You also need to eliminate cola drinks, chocolate, tea, cakes and biscuits from your diet, at least in the hours leading up to bed time.

It is also a mistake to try to use alcohol to help you get off to sleep, because although it may appear to do the trick it actually destroys the B vitamins important for maintaining normal sleep rhythms.

Irritable Bowel Syndrome

Irritable Bowel Syndrome, or IBS, which affects an estimated quarter of the adult population and twice as many women as men, is now the leading cause of absenteeism after the common cold. The symptoms, which include stomach cramps, typically alternate between constipation and diarrhoea, making it a condition people don't like talking about and leaving too many suffering in silence. There's another good reason to tackle this problem as soon as it starts – if you ignore it, it will only get worse and can lead to more serious conditions such as colitis.

The good news is that there is plenty you can do, and most of it is as simple as avoiding the foods known to exacerbate the problem. Two-thirds of IBS sufferers, for example, have been found to have hidden food intolerances. The worst culprits are wheat, dairy, coffee, tea, citrus fruits and lactose (the sugar in cow's milk).

You may also hear health practitioners talk about something called Dysbiosis – this is the name given to an imbalance of the bacteria in the digestive tract which, in the right proportions, promote good health and easy digestion. When this balance is disturbed, IBS can take hold. Other causes include too much stress, too little fibre in the diet, too much junk food (which overburdens the liver), and too much alcohol or other stimulants which tax the whole system. Eating live yoghurt may help, but you won't always know which strains of live bacteria you're eating. Probiotic supplements do a much better job, providing high levels of the Bifidobacteria which, in the right proportions, will alleviate constipation and prevent diarrhoea.

Natural probiotics include bananas, onions, garlic, artichokes, barley, rye, tomatoes, honey and asparagus, but if you already have IBS you can't really eat enough to make a big difference. Cut out stimulants including tea, coffee, alcohol and chocolate, and avoid wheat, dairy and citrus fruits. Substitute soya or even goats' milk for cow's milk. Your symptoms should improve over six months, after which you can start to re-introduce the offending foods in small quantities. If symptoms recur, eliminate them again. Find a way to reduce stress – maybe take up yoga, tai chi or autogenic training.

Many IBS sufferers are found to be lacking in the B vitamins so need to take a good B complex supplement. You should also be taking a probiotic supplement such as *Lactobacillus acidophilus*. This will rebuild levels of friendly bacteria in your gut in a more controlled way. Feed these replacement bacteria by supplementing your diet with the Fructo-oligosaccharides (the name is always shortened to FOS) which act as a fast food for all those beneficial bacteria that help digestion. A complex sugar, derived from plants, FOS taste sweet like sugar but act in the body like fibre because they have a molecular structure which passes, undigested, from the stomach to the large intestine. Sold as either a powder or a syrup, make sure the brand you buy is at least 95% pure.

Magnesium is the second-most common deficiency in men and woman, yet it is crucial for proper bowel functioning. If you supplement it, you need to take calcium as well, in a ratio of 2:1 in favour of the calcium.

Aloe vera juice is the IBS sufferer's nectar. It soothes and heals the damaged lining of the gut when you drink enough of it. Make sure the brand you buy is high in the mucopolysaccharides (the active ingredients). Drink a quarter of a glass in the morning and again at night. I also recommend nettle tea. This is an acquired taste but an excellent liver tonic which will also stimulate the digestive tract. Try and drink three cups of an organic brand every day.

Leaky Gut

In a healthy gut, the lining of the intestines generates new cells faster than any other tissue in the body. When working properly, these cells form a semi-permeable lining, which acts like a filter, allowing essential nutrients to pass through but blocking toxins and other nutrients, which may cause an allergic reaction if they get into the bloodstream.

Damage to the intestinal lining – usually caused by junk diets, alcohol, bacterial or parasite infections and prescription drugs – can increase the permeability, giving rise to a condition known as Leaky Gut. This is now believed to be at the root of many auto-immune diseases, including inflammatory bowel and arthritis. Researchers have also found higher gut permeability in both children and adults suffering from asthma and eczema than in those not suffering these conditions. Candida also increases gut permeability.

Anthony Haynes, the award-winning clinical nutritionist and founder of The Nutrition Clinic in London, says 80% of his clients are suffering some kind of digestive disorder at the start of treatment. This is, of course, a self-selecting group, but there is no question that increased gut permeability has now been linked with Crohn's disease, food allergies, Coeliac disease, chronic skin complaints, rheumatoid arthritis and other inflammatory joint conditions, as well as neurological imbalances and Chronic Fatigue. As Anthony Haynes says:

'The lining of your gut is thinner than an eyelid. It takes just four days to regenerate itself and over a lifetime, it will help process 25 tonnes of food. It is far more sensitive and permeable than your skin and is the true interface between your body and the outside world.'

Once a Leaky Gut has developed, the regular consumption of everyday foods can cause an allergic and inflammatory response. These frequently include wheat, dairy, citrus fruits, eggs, chickens and peanuts. Aloe Vera juice, which we know is rich in substances called mucopolysaccharides, soothes and heals the lining of the intestine. Again, nettle tea – an excellent liver and digestive tonic – can also help.

A deficiency in zinc, which is essential for a healthy immune response to inflammation caused by food allergens, may exacerbate the problem. Vitamin A, which helps repair the body's membrane linings, including the gut, is also important. You can drink cabbage water, which is used in the treatment of ulcers, and a nutritionist may also suggest taking a supplement of quercetin, a bioflavanoid which has been shown to help reduce inflammation. You can ask your nutritionist to book a gut permeability urine test. This should cost in the region of £60 and will determine the extent of the problem.

Liver Regeneration

Raw eggs contain an amino acid called N-acetyl-cysteine (NAC), which has been shown to improve liver function in human and animal studies. It is frequently included in hangover remedies and works by boosting levels of a compound called glutathione, which helps the body clear toxins from alcohol and cigarette smoking. In one study, reported in the *Medical Journal of Australia* in 1980, 11 patients who were at risk of liver damage following serious paracetamol poisoning were given injections of NAC. The results showed complete regeneration of the liver with no reported side-effects.

If in the past you have been a heavy drinker, you would benefit from daily supplements of an incredible herb called milk thistle. Popular with European herbalists, this is one of the safest of all the herbal remedies and again, regenerates damaged liver cells.

The active ingredient is silymarin, which is extracted from the seeds. It works by altering the outer membrane of liver cells so toxins cannot penetrate the organ. Better still, it stimulates the production of a chemical called RNA polymerase A, which boosts ribosome protein synthesis to regenerate the liver. The recommended dosage is 200–400mg of the active ingredient daily.

Please remember, though, that herbs can be as potent as prescription drugs and may interfere with other medication. Do not self-dose for such a serious condition, but find a qualified medical herbalist who can help.

Lupus Disease

An auto-immune disease which can cause either recurring red round patches of skin rash (discoid lupus) or inflammation in joints, tendons, connective tissue and other organs (systemic lupus), this condition affects mostly young women in their late teens to 30s. Auto-immune simply means that instead of protecting the body, the immune system attacks it. The conventional treatment is steroids, which suppress this aberrant immune activity.

There is often a family history of this disease, which can also be triggered by environmental pollution. Risk factors include suffering from asthma, low blood levels of antioxidants, especially vitamins A and E, and having irregular periods. In most sufferers, sunlight has been shown to be the usual trigger of the first-ever outbreak of discoid lupus.

There have been reports of people improving after switching to a vegetarian diet and, according to early studies, you may benefit from cutting out foods which are high in phenylalanine (chocolate, apples, chicken and peanuts) and tyrosine (dairy products, fish and oats). Foods that are high in the omega-3 fatty acids, especially fish and flaxseed (linseed), have been shown to reduce lupus inflammation too.

Many sufferers are intolerant of dairy products, especially cow's milk – which contains casein, a protein that has immune-stimulating properties.

Smoking definitely increases the risk, although, somewhat unusually, drinking alcohol decreases it. Selenium, another antioxidant, has helped clear lupus in animals and there is early evidence that for those with the discoid form, vitamin E can help.

Pantothenic acid (vitamin B_5) is also worth investigating. In one study, 67 people with discoid lupus took 10–15mg per day, along with 1,500–3,000 iu of vitamin E for 19 months; they reported significant improvements.

Herbalists recommend herbs such as clivers and yellow dock to improve the lymphatic system (which drains away toxins), and gentian to boost good digestion and encourage feelings of greater well-being. These herbs will also help the liver and the kidneys with the elimination of the body's waste matter.

Herbs which can help relax and tone the nervous system, such as hops and hypericum (St John's Wort), will also be beneficial for overall well-being and the condition of your skin.

Please note that alfalfa has been linked with worsening this condition. It contains L-canavanine which can trigger an auto-immune response in susceptible individuals.

Menopause

The best-kept secret of good health during menopause is to eat as naturally as possible. Researchers have found, for example, that it is better to eat smaller but more frequent meals, which will help stabilise blood sugar levels, and to try to avoid tea, coffee, refined sugar and alcohol, which not only disrupt these levels but which also deprive the body of vital nutrients.

The drop in oestrogen levels which occurs during menopause is believed to leave women more at risk of osteoporosis and cardiovascular disease, so as well as treating menopausal symptoms, vitamins and herbs can also be useful in protecting against these other two conditions.

Moderate exercise will build bone strength – just 50 skips a day can increase bone density by a small but significant 4%. Eating foods that are rich in phyto-estrogens which help rebalance hormones, will also help. Tofu and organic soya are two good examples. (In Japanese, there is no equivalent phrase to describe the menopausal 'hot flush'.)

Exercise can also reduce stress, which is another trigger for some of the worst symptoms of menopause, including those dreaded flushes. You need a diet that is rich in the B vitamins – known as nature's own stress-busters – which cannot be stored in the body but must be replaced every day. Good healthy food sources of these important nutrients include poultry, salmon, eggs, almonds, cheese, bran, brown rice and yoghurt.

Another important nutrient is magnesium, the second-most commonly deficient mineral in women. Known as nature's tranquilliser and found in brown pasta, nuts and pulses, it also plays a key role in the absorption of calcium, which will help protect against osteoporosis during menopause. If you supplement either of these nutrients, you will affect levels of the other. This is known as synergy. The ideal ratio here is 2:1 in favour of the calcium. So, if you take 500mg of calcium, take 250mg of magnesium too.

The nutrients most lacking in the Western diet are the omega-3 fatty acids, which work wonders for many women during menopause. They help the body make substances called prostaglandins which then regulate hormones, decrease blood pressure and reduce water retention. These chemicals also reduce the stickiness of blood platelets which, in turn, helps prevent heart attacks and strokes.

The body cannot make the omega-3 fatty acids but must get them from the diet. They enhance the immune system, boost energy and soften the skin. You can increase your dietary intake by eating more cold water oily fish such as mackerel, pilchards, herring and sardines or investigate their availability in supplements.

Long before people had access to qualified doctors, the wise herb women in villages and towns (who were often the local midwives, too) knew just what herbs to prescribe for everyday ailments. Many of these remedies, which have an excellent track record in treating menopausal symptoms, are enjoying renewed popularity today.

The most effective herbs during menopause are those that help to rebalance hormone levels. These have what is known as adaptogenic properties and include Agnus castus (or chaste berry), which can help prevent hot flushes for many women. Valerian is used to ease tension, and Korean (Panax) Ginseng will boost the activities of the adrenal glands, which sit on top of the kidneys and which produce adrenaline in response to stress signals from the body.

Sage will relieve hot flushes but if you have to choose just one herb to ease you through what is, after all, a perfectly natural rite of passage, then take the strange-sounding Chinese herb dong quai, which has oestrogenic properties and which nourishes and thickens the thinned walls of the vagina and bladder. This thinning is perfectly natural but may, at first, trigger cystitis. Dong quai can also help ease menopausal rheumatism and is rich in magnesium, to deepen sleep disturbed by night sweats.

During times of stress and change, the liver, which is the body's main detoxification organ, can become overburdened. Some of the work of the ovaries is taken on by the hormone-controlling adrenal glands, and these too can become overburdened. To support these systems you should think about taking dandelion, which can help re-regulate hormones during menopause and which will also act to decongest the liver. You can eat the young leaves in a salad or take a herbal tincture.

Kitty Campion, the medical herbalist and author of *Menopause Naturally*, describes hormone replacement therapy (HRT), as 'the biggest medical bungle of the 21st century'. She says herbs and nutrition are enough to help every woman through the menopause.

Many women have also discovered so-called menopausal 'cakes'. More like a heavy fruit loaf, these are packed with nutrients to smooth your passage through the menopause. They can be expensive, though. For details of how to make your own, contact The Women's Nutritional Advisory Service (see Resources).

Warning: If you have any underlying health problem or if you are already taking medication, consult your doctor before changing your diet or taking herbs. If you are taking antidepressants or tranquillisers, do not take Korean Ginseng. If taking HRT, do not take dong quai. To find a medical herbalist who can determine the right combination of herbs for you, see Resources.

Male Menopause

Much has been written about the female menopause, HRT and various alternatives for women, but very little about the idea of a similar transitional period in men's lives. Men, like women, do suffer a gradual decline in levels of sex hormones as they age and, increasingly, doctors are considering the idea of a male menopause. The theory is that, as with menopausal woman, these fluctuations in hormone levels may be responsible for a reduction in bone density, muscle wasting and loss of libido too. It follows, then, that these could be combatted by testosterone replacement therapy, although this, like female HRT, will have unwelcome side-effects in some men. Too much testosterone, for example, has been linked with prostate problems, so it makes sense to investigate more natural remedies, at least at the outset.

Lots of companies now make general multivitamin supplements formulated specifically for men with all the vitamins and minerals you may be lacking if you are in your middle years. You need to take one that includes zinc, which is of crucial importance to reproductive health in men. There are also two important herbal remedies that will further ease your passage through the male menopause. Saw palmetto, which is used in many prostate-protecting preparations, actually has a balancing effect on hormones and, as well as helping boost low hormone levels, will revert excess levels to normal. Buy it in organic tincture form and take as directed on the bottle.

To support your libido, herbalists recommend a herb called damiana which is a small, aromatic shrub that is native to South America where it is known for its aphrodisiac properties. Described as a stimulant tonic for the reproductive organs in both sexes, it is also used for impotence, sterility and anxiety in men.

In Japan, men suffer the same rates of prostate cancers as Westerners but mortality rates are much lower. Researchers now suggest that this is due to the high levels of phytoestrogens in the diet, which can help to rebalance hormones naturally in both sexes. To benefit from these compounds, step up your intake of soya, chickpeas and lentils.

The only way to prevent a loss of bone density is to take more exercise. Use it or lose it, as they say. A 30-minute daily walk can keep bones strong, and just five minutes of skipping each day has been shown to improve bone density in women by 4%. This may not sound much, but it can make the difference between skeletal strength and vulnerability.

Migraines

For years, chocolate has topped the list of the common food triggers believed to cause migraine-type headache, but new research by scientists at the University of Pittsburgh's Pain Evaluation and Treatment Institute turns conventional thinking on its head by suggesting this is not necessarily so.

In an illuminating study, 63 women, all suffering from chronic headaches and 50% suffering from migraines, first followed a special diet which restricted their intake of amine (the substance found in chocolate and other foods including dates, citrus fruits, yeast, nuts, dairy products and red wine), which are believed to cause headaches. Each participant then underwent double-blind clinical trials in which they were given two samples of chocolate and two of carob, in random order. They all kept diaries monitoring diet and headaches. The researchers concluded that, despite the women's own beliefs about chocolate causing headaches, it was no more of a culprit than carob.

Nutritionists claim food triggers are responsible for up to 90% of migraine cases, but even they accept it is difficult for a sufferer to identify exactly which foods they are reacting to. One woman, for example, discovered her headaches were triggered by cinnamon, which is unlikely to be on the list of foods the doctor suggests you avoid. Elimination and rotation diets can help pinpoint more obvious culprits, but the task is also made more problematic by the fact that it can take more than a week for your system to react to a particular food you may have eaten.

Also, no two migraines are the same, according to Penny Povey, a medical herbalist who practises at Farmacia in London. She frequently treats women, for example, who suffer migraines caused by hormonal disturbances around the time of menstruation and which are so severe, they spend three days in bed vomiting. Many sufferers will recognise her description of flashing lights and the desperate need to retreat to somewhere quiet and dark.

Homeopathy, which has proven highly effective for many sufferers, keys in to these differences and makes a point of prescribing remedies according not only to the type of pain but how it starts. If the headache is worse on the right side, for example, and if trying to concentrate makes the pain worse, your homoeopath is likely to suggest Lycopodium 6c. Blurring of the vision and vomiting would suggest Iris 6c, while a throbbing, blinding headache with a feeling of congestion in the head would probably be best treated by Natrum mur. 6c.

Whatever the type of pain, the herb feverfew has an excellent track record in helping to keep migraines at bay when taken daily. It can take up to a month to kick in, so you need to persevere. Take 50 drops of an organic tincture with your breakfast each morning. Please note, however, that you must not take feverfew if you are already taking warfarin or during pregnancy.

A qualified herbalist can also tailor-make a remedy to take as soon as you sense the onset of a migraine. This is likely to include a mild sedative such as valerian, which first appeared in the US *Pharmacopoeia* as a tranquilliser in 1820.

In another American study by scientists at the University of Cincinnati College of Medicine, taking fish oil capsules daily was shown not only to halve the number of migraine attacks but to reduce the pain and the severity of those that did occur. In the trial, 60% of subjects benefited from the supplement, which reduced the number of attacks from two a week to two a fortnight. Men reported more relief than women. If you are going to investigate this nutritional approach, make sure you are taking fish oils made from an unpolluted source.

Many sufferers have been found to be deficient in magnesium, but Gareth Zeal, nutritional advisor to the GNC retail chain, says you need to take a pretty hefty dose – 2x500mg tablets daily – to benefit. Vitamin B_2 has also been shown to help reduce the number of attacks, and as the B vitamins work best when taken together, take a balanced B complex supplement plus another supplement to provide the equivalent of 400mg of B_2 daily.

The immediate cause of a migraine headache is a constriction and then a swelling of the arteries which supply the brain. Why this should suddenly happen between the ages of 10 and 30, and why these attacks are three times more common in women than men, is anybody's guess – although abnormally low levels of the neurotransmitter serotonin have been identified in sufferers. In women, the contraceptive pill has also been linked with migraines.

There is strong evidence of a genetic risk – if one parent is a sufferer then a child has a 40% chance of getting migraines too – but they can also disappear in middle age, as suddenly as they started which for those who are still suffering is one good reason to look forward to getting older.

Mi-Gon is a roll-on herbal remedy with near-miraculous powers. It was developed by David Evans, a sufferer who was then able to reduce his migraine medication by 80% over 12 months. It contains peppermint and sweet basil oils, both of which have analgesic properties (see Resources).

Mood-Boosters

Scientists have now identified some 40 brain chemicals or neurotransmitters. Serotonin is probably the best known of all these. It is linked with sleep patterns (see Insomnia, page 173), mood and perception. Too little may cause sleeplessness and depression. Too much has been linked with premature ageing, psychosis and aggression.

The brain makes serotonin from a common amino acid called tryptophan, which can be found in foods such as spinach, cauliflower, broccoli, bananas, cottage cheese, fennel, fish, sweet potatoes, turkey, soybeans, chicken and watercress. To enhance the transport of tryptophan across the blood-brain barrier – which only allows oxygen, glucose and a few selected nutrients to pass through – you need to step up your intake of carbohydrates. These cause the pancreas to make more insulin, which in turn gets rid of other amino acids which would otherwise compete with tryptophan to reach the brain. Tryptophan, then, is needed to make serotonin, and what you buy in supplement form is a derivative called 5-hydroxy-tryptophan or 5-HTP.

The chemical linked with the 'high' of being in love is called phenylethylalanine. Once passion starts to fade, the brain stops its output of this chemical, which is derived from phenylalanine – an amino acid found in many common foods including chocolate. This explains why the lovelorn will reach for the chocolate box when an affair ends. Other foods that are rich natural sources of phenylalanine include almonds, apples, carrots, chicken, peanuts, pineapples, eggs, tomatoes, beetroot, herring and milk.

Stimulants such as tea and coffee and refined sugar can all rapidly elevate blood sugar levels and then cause an equally rapid slump. This is the biochemical cause of fluctuating moods, unexplained tiredness and irritability. It also explains why people feel better after that first cup of coffee in the morning. Caffeine stimulates the release of adrenaline, which, in turn, raises blood sugar levels to make you feel more alert and energetic. The slump that follows, which leaves you feeling ratty and sluggish, is, sadly, inevitable.

If you feel irritable and tired for no reason, you need to start changing your diet in ways that will help regulate your blood sugar levels to improve your mood. Avoid the refined sugars, which you now know can cause fluctuations, and when you do eat, make sure you combine a little protein, fibre and carbohydrate at every meal.

For a mood-improving breakfast, for example, try a bowl of unsweetened yoghurt with fresh fruit, or have a couple of poached eggs on rye toast. In winter, oat bran porridge provides a steady release of energy. Both these meals will provide a steady release of glucose, which means more consistent energy for you. Stay away from caffeine; try organic herbal teas instead.

Eating smaller meals more frequently should also help avoid the wild fluctuations that are making you bad-tempered. A small snack at bedtime, say some fruit and cottage cheese, will help keep blood sugar levels stabilised throughout the night.

You may also benefit from taking a supplement of chromium, which works with insulin in the metabolism of sugar. Take a maximum of 300 micrograms a day – 200 of which you should take last thing at night to improve your mood when you awake. Even better, Biotics Research make a combination supplement called Glucobalance which does just what the name suggests. It contains all the anti-stress B vitamins, the antioxidant A, C and E vitamins plus chromium, selenium, magnesium and zinc. Take two with your breakfast and two again at bedtime. For suppliers, see Resources.

Morning Tiredness

Morning tiredness can be a sign of any one of a number of nutritional problems, from a straightforward deficiency in one or more nutrients to poor digestion, an overburdened liver, food intolerance or a blood sugar imbalance. The latter is the most common cause and is usually the result of a diet that is too high in refined, processed foods and in too many stimulants such as tea, coffee and alcohol.

Your tiredness could also be the result of a deficiency in any of the vitamins and minerals which are crucial for the production of glucose, which the body converts to energy in the cell. These include the B vitamins, magnesium, chromium, zinc, vitamin C, iron and coenzyme Q10.

The solution is to start a supplementation regime taking a good quality multivitamin and -mineral with 200mcg of chromium and 50mg of coenzyme Q10. Cut out refined foods, tea, coffee, alcohol and sugar and introduce more fibre into your diet from natural sources such as whole grains, beans, lentils, nuts, seeds, raw fruits and vegetables.

If these changes do not produce a significant improvement, consult a qualified nutritionist who can determine if you suffer food intolerances, poor digestion and/or poor liver functioning (or even overwork) and treat you accordingly.

Nails

Holistic practitioners seldom agree on the reason for many nail problems. Some believe herbs and vitamins can help. Others say most of the conditions that affect nails are caused by a lack of oxygen, linked to lung conditions, and that nutrition is unlikely to help. The one thing they do all agree on is that the nails can be an important mirror to your health and reveal what is happening internally.

The B vitamins are known to strengthen animal hooves, and although nobody knows why or how this happens, Swiss researchers decided to see if the same held true for humans. They gave 2.5mg of biotin (one of the B vitamins) every day to women complaining of brittle nails. After six months, their nail thickness had increased by 25%. In another study, 63% of Americans taking similar quantities of biotin each day showed a significant improvement in the condition of their nails, and a reduction in splitting.

There remains little specific research in this area, but I have heard very strong anecdotal evidence that organic sulphur supplements will also help. Designed originally as an anti-inflammatory to help relieve joint and muscle problems, Methyl Sulphonyl Methane, sold as MSM, can improve the condition of your hair and nails. It is a naturally-occurring form of sulphur that is found in many raw foods and rainwater, but we rarely get enough of it in our diets because it is destroyed by cooking and food-processing techniques. Levels also drop off as we age. It is present in keratin – the tough substance that makes up nails – and is also crucial for collagen, the main component of the body's connective tissues.

Many health practitioners will examine the condition as well as the strength of your nails, to gain an insight into your general state of health. White spots, for example, have long been seen as a sign of zinc deficiency in Traditional Chinese Medicine. Ridges, especially horizontal ones, and flaking nails are often interpreted as a sign of vitamin and mineral deficiencies, especially the B vitamins already mentioned, iron, silica, calcium and sulphur (as before). They may also point to insufficient protein in the diet, although this would be unusual in the West, unless there is also an underlying eating disorder.

The herb horsetail is a rich source of silica and will be used by herbalists and homeopaths to help prevent brittle nails. Researchers have found that calcium alone is not as effective as it is when there is enough silica present, which is another example of the synergy mentioned at the beginning of this section. Dandelions are so packed with nutrients they can help improve the condition of the nails when anaemia and an iron deficiency are the underlying cause. Alfalfa, once called the father of all herbs, is also used to help build the blood. It is believed to contain all the vitamins and minerals known to man, and is high in vitamin D, which enhances the absorption of calcium in the body.

Osteoarthritis

Probably the most common of all the joint diseases, osteoarthritis is believed to affect up to a third of the 45- to 65-year-old age group and 75% of those older than this. It affects the hips, knees or spine, and the primary cause is the degeneration of the joint cartilage which should both protect the joint and enable bones to move without friction. When cartilage is worn away, it leaves the bone endings exposed, which can then cause pain, stiffness and deformities (including swelling) of the joints.

Glucosamine is a natural component of cartilage. It stimulates the production of connective tissue in the body, but as we get older we cannot make enough of it naturally. In some studies, glucosamine has been shown to halt the progress of osteoarthritis by tackling the underlying cause and restoring lost cartilage. So, while anti-inflammatory drugs will act faster, glucosamine is more effective over time. In addition, it is safe and has no side-effects except in rare cases where it may cause nausea or heartburn; even this can be countered by taking it with food.

David Wilkie, the Olympic swimming champion – in 1976, he was the first British male swimmer for 68 years to win an Olympic title when he set a world record of 2:15,11 in the 200m breaststroke – is now the managing director of Health Perception, the company which first brought glucosamine to Europe back in 1989. He says he first began taking the supplement in his twenties to relieve a bad back when he was training in America. He has seen sales rocket by 300% since launching glucosamine formulated with vitamin C and with bone-building calcium in the UK, and says the supplement has also become hugely popular with sportsmen and -women anxious to get back to their sport after suffering an injury.

One problem, now the supplement has become so popular, is that because there is a fast buck to be made from selling cheaper versions, the market has frequently been flooded with inferior products in which the dosage has not been standardised. This would also explain why you may hear conflicting reports as to the efficacy of glucosamine. Also, you will not feel the benefits immediately but may have to take it for three months to see a significant improvement. So if you do decide to try it, check you are taking glucosamine SO4 which works and not glucosamine UC1 which is much cheaper but which does not work.

Ozone Therapy

Ozone (O_3) is a clear blue gas which has been described as the best bactericide, fungicide and viricide known to man – but only by those who swear by it. The American Food and Drug Administration (FDA), maintains it has no therapeutic benefits, yet in Germany alone, some 7,000 doctors offer it to their patients.

Lately there has been much talk of its possible benefit in the treatment of cancer – particularly cancer of the breast – but I have come across some very dubious fly-by-night companies spouting pseudo-science and offering this treatment. According to the FDA, the treatment is downright fraudulent. What is clear is that we need more research.

The theory, in the treatment of cancer, is that the ozone inhibits tumour metabolism and boosts the activity of the body's own defences, the phagocytes, which also produce hydroxyl to kill bacteria and viruses. Ozone is also said to oxidise the outer lipid layer of malignant cells and destroy them by a process known as lysis – which means it disintegrates them.

As well as activating and strengthening the immune system by increasing the amount of interferon produced, ozone is also said to boost oxygen levels in the bloodstream, which then bolsters overall health.

There are practitioners who specialise in offering this treatment, but be careful whom you see. There are no accredited training schemes, which means anyone can buy the equipment and go into business. This is, of course, one of the main reasons the treatment remains so controversial. Another reason it may not have won over many devotees is that in some clinics the ozone is administered either via the rectum or intravaginally. If you are shy or remotely self-conscious about your body, this is unlikely to be a therapy you would be in any rush to try out.

Panic Attacks

Hypnotherapy, in the hands of a skilled practitioner, is one of the fastest and most effective ways of treating anxiety attacks, which are the physical symptoms of extreme emotional stress. If you are a sufferer, see your condition as a kind of wake-up call designed to get you to make an honest appraisal of your life and the way you are living it. Sufferers often have a history of a past loss, for example, which has not been properly processed. One of the advantages of hypnosis is that you will unravel the underlying cause. You will also be taught self-help technqiues which will help you stay calm when you feel an attack threatening.

The other good thing about hypnotherapy is that it can be a very positive adjunct to any other therapy or treatment you are already having. You should not need more than 3-5 sessions with a reputable practitioner, and may even be back in control after just one.

Remember, your session will only be as good as the hypnotherapist. If you cannot get a word-of-mouth recommendation from a trusted friend, find a practitioner through one of the accredited governing bodies (see Resources.) If you come out of your first session uncertain about whether you have, indeed, been hypnotised, don't bother going back (some estimates suggest only 10% of the population are deep trance subjects). With a skilled practitioner you will feel safe and comfortable through the session but you will also be in no doubt that you have entered a very deep form of relaxation allowing your subconscious to be reached.

If you suffer from nervousness and general anxiety, homeopathy and the Bach Flower Remedies will help (see Resources to find a practitioner). You will also benefit from Kava Kava tincture. This herb, which has now become quite fashionable, has been used for years by Polynesian healers. It contains kavalactones, which promote calmness and tranquillity, acting on the limbic or most ancient part of the brain. This controls all other brain activities and is the principal seat of your emotions.

Parasites

Parasitic infections are not only a hazard when you are travelling but can take hold even when you stay at home. 40% of children under the age of 10, for example, have threadworms, no matter how clean their home.

If you are planning to travel, the best way to prevent catching any of the organisms which can cause a severe stomach upset and, even worse, long-term health problems is to embark on an antiparasitic, antifungal treatment a month before you plan to depart, and to continue with the treatment for a month after your return.

Alison Loftus, a nutritionist who specialises in parasite infections, started this programme by taking a herb called *Artemesia*, which not only aids digestion but also maintains the natural balance of the flora in the intestinal tract. Take this as a tincture and aim for the equivalent of 1g a day. You should also take 300mg a day of *berberis* which, as well as flushing out toxins, regulating digestion and improving bowel function, will also support immune function. You can further boost your immunity by taking vitamin A (7,500iu); vitamin C (1g) and vitamin E (100iu), plus 25mcg of selenium and 15mg of zinc, daily.

Both grapefruit extract (Citricidal) and garlic are antibacterial, antifungal and antiparasitic agents and are effective against a wide range of parasites and bacteria.

To tackle any existing parasitic infection, a three-pronged attack is needed. First, you have to kill off the organism, then expel it and finally, take steps to prevent re-infection. When treating children, grapefruit seed extract is more palatable when taken in a non-acidic fruit juice such as apple. Also, avoid sugar in the diet until the treatment ends.

For adults, there are many herbs that can help. Black walnut is a favourite among herbalists, who use it, for example, to kill off worms. False unicorn will help expel them, while ground pumpkin seeds, sprinkled on your cereal, will do both jobs fast. Horsetail kills off both the parasite and its eggs, and garlic contains sulphur, which is also deadly for such infections although not a favourite with children.

Polycystic Ovarian Syndrome (PCOS)

If you spend an hour a week secretly tweezing out unwanted facial hair, if you bloat and gain weight even on the strictest calorie-controlled diet, if you escaped the curse of teenage acne but woke up one morning to the horror of your adult face erupting and if you have been trying, unsuccessfully, to get pregnant for years, you are likely to be suffering from a miserable condition that affects as many as one in five women – most of whom will not know they have it.

Polycystic Ovarian Syndrome (PCOS) is a serious underlying hormonal imbalance that for years has been masked by symptoms which women suffer in silent embarrassment or unwittingly present to the wrong people – the beautician or dermatologist – to treat. Few doctors have the time or the experience to link this litany of seemingly irritating but trivial complaints to reach a diagnosis, and those that do have been trained to prescribe Dianette – a combination of oestrogen with progesterone, which, it is now shown, will only make the condition worse.

For many sufferers, PCOS is only diagnosed when an ultrasound scan to investigate unexplained infertility shows a string of tiny, fluid-filled cysts laced across the ovaries, looking for all the world like a pearl necklace. The result of a major hormone imbalance and too much testosterone in the body, PCOS is an inherited condition and there is no known cure. The symptoms themselves may not appear life-threatening, but the overall risks associated with having it are much higher than doctors previously thought.

A woman with PCOS is, according to new research, 7 times more likely to develop diabetes than a woman of the same age and lifestyle who does not have the syndrome. She is also now known to be 7.4 more times at risk of a heart attack and 4 times more likely to suffer from high blood pressure. The first two of these conditions are major killers in the Western world, which is why, finally, PCOS is getting the attention it deserves.

One of the reasons it is so difficult for doctors and health practitioners to recognise and diagnose is that this endocrine disorder can vary wildly in its severity. In its worst form, it causes obesity and hirsutism – but again, only 50% of sufferers will present with these telltale signs.

Dr Adam Carey, a reproductive endocrinologist and co-founder of the Centre for Nutritional Medicine in London, is also the co-author of the first book dedicated to PCOS, yet even he admits that when he worked in hospitals he would prescribe Dianette for women presenting with the symptoms of PCOS. This, it is now known, not only fails to tackle the underlying condition but will actually make it worse. The symptoms will improve over the short-term, say 2–3 years, but when they return, they are likely to be even more severe.

The two key biochemical markers of PCOS are that sufferers make too much insulin and too much testosterone. Researchers are now certain the two are linked, and a study published in the US journal *Proceedings of the National Academy of Sciences* has suggested this link is a gene called follistain which has two telltale functions: It plays a role in the development of the ovaries and it is needed to make insulin.

Testosterone, which is believed to be made by these tiny ovarian cysts, is carried in the bloodstream by a substance called sex hormone binding globulin SHBG. Think of SHBG as a car transporter without which runaway or 'free' testosterone molecules bind in the wrong places, including under the skin where they cause acne and excess facial hair. One of the symptoms of PCOS is a tendency to put on weight, and when your weight increases, the amount of SHBG, which is made by the liver, decreases. This explains why reducing your weight is so crucial in controlling and even reversing PCOS.

Insulin works to control sugar levels in the blood but women with PCOS are known to be resistant to their own insulin. It is, says Dr Carey, as if the cells have gone deaf and can no longer pick up messages from the pancreas, which makes insulin, about how much is needed. When this system breaks down the body reacts by storing more of the calories from your food, especially carbohydrates, as fat. You put on weight, even though you are eating the same amount. Excess insulin also acts on the ovaries to make more testosterone, which is the very last thing you need.

You can manage the symptoms and help reverse PCOS by changing your diet to eat less carbohydrate and to eat smaller, more frequent meals. This will avoid sudden rushes of blood sugar and so help control insulin production and prevent weight gain. Protein has been shown to reduce the rate of glucose absorption and stabilise insulin production, so eat a little protein with each meal. Cut out refined carbohydrates, which means all cakes and biscuits, and take exercise to maintain your optimum weight.

The biochemistry of PCOS is fascinating, but even more gripping, says Dr Carey, is the realisation that here is a genetic condition which, although there is no cure, sufferers can manage through diet and lifestyle changes: 'It is a condition where women really can use their environment to interact with their genetic programming and create a positive outcome.'

For those seeking an alternative approach in addition to nutritional changes, Traditional Chinese Medicine reports fantastic results treating hormonal disturbances including PCOS. Practitioner Zita West, a former NHS midwife who specialises in holistic health for women, has helped many PCOS sufferers conceive through a combination of acupuncture and rebalancing herbal and vitamin supplements.

She knows that, to many Westerners, the idea of auricular (ear) acupuncture sounds bonkers, but she claims – and there is plenty of anecdotal evidence to support this – that it is a powerful tool to help with conception when the underlying problem is one of hormones gone haywire:

'Rebalancing hormones is part of our Wellbeing Programme where we like to treat a woman on a weekly basis. Traditional Chinese Medicine, for example, pays particular attention to the body's energy channels and centres and I have noticed, with a lot of women suffering from PCOS, that the lower channels are very cold.'

According to Zita, this is easily remedied using a technique called moxibustion where, instead of needles, the practitioner uses a herb which is a form of mugwort. This is shaped into small cones and placed at the appropriate acupuncture points before being warmed with a flame. It does not hurt but actually creates a very soothing warmth throughout the body as it stimulates a revitalised energy flow.

Pregnancy

Most women know to start taking folic acid (at least 400mcg per day) even before they conceive to reduce the risk of spinal tube defects in their baby, but there are other supplements and herbs that can also help keep mother and baby well. Evening primrose oil, for example, will keep the skin supple and prevent stretch marks. It can also protect against 'Brain Fog' – that peculiar feeling of vagueness which affects lots of women in later pregnancy when the baby is leeching all the essential fatty acids from the mother's diet.

A less well-known substance which does the same is docosahexanoic acid, a fish oil whose name is thankfully shortened to DHA. This is vital for the development of the baby, especially during the last trimester when there is rapid growth of the child's brain. The baby cannot make its own DHA and so, again, gets its supply from the mother. Vitamin B_6 can help prevent stretch marks and zinc too, is important, especially if you know you are having a boy, since a male child takes five times more zinc from the mother's diet than a girl.

A good general multivitamin and -mineral is important during pregnancy, but it makes sense to use one that is formulated specifically for women. Zita West, a former NHS midwife and acupuncturist who now specialises in Traditional Chinese Medicine (TCM), has formulated an excellent mail-order range for mothers-to-be which includes a multisupplement powder called Pregvital and DHA capsules, and which deserves to be better known (see Resources).

Since pregnancy is a time when most mothers want to avoid drug treatments, acupuncture is a popular alternative, especially for the relief of morning sickness, vomiting, backache, headaches and sciatica. A lot of women find it useful during labour, too.

Prostate Protection

Since it is obvious to me that lots of people, including and especially men, do not know very much about the prostate gland, we will take a look at what it is and what it does before examining which nutrients and herbs can help to keep it healthy.

The prostate is a small gland that surrounds the neck of the bladder and urethra (the tube that carries urine from the bladder) in men. It is the size of a grain of rice at birth, but grows to walnut-size in adulthood when its job is to contribute to the seminal fluid, which carries the sperm.

If this gland begins to swell and enlarge, usually because of hormone changes associated with ageing, it puts pressure on the urethra. This is the condition known as Benign Prostatic Hyperplasia (BPH), which some estimates claim affects half of all men aged 50, and 80% of those in their eighties. The symptoms include needing to urinate more often, straining to pass water, and having less control over this process, especially dribbling at the end. At its most severe, this condition can make it impossible to urinate and will cause a urinary tract infection that could lead to kidney failure. Drugs can help, but at least one of those prescribed (finasteride) causes impotence. The better news is that herbs and nutrients can do the same job without the nasty side-effects.

In one recent trial, men taking 159mcg a day of selenium had three times less risk of developing prostate problems than those taking just 86mcg a day. Daily zinc supplements (at least 15mg a day) have also helped the prostate return to near normal in 70% of sufferers who agreed to take part in a trial that continued over several months. As far back as 1941, 19 men who were given essential fatty acid (EFA) supplements all reported an improved libido, a reduction in the enlargement of the prostate and, for the majority of those taking part, a cessation of the urge to urinate during the night. We still need more research with larger numbers, but one tablespoon of flaxseed oil a day will make sure you are getting enough EFAs. Since these also increase the demand for vitamin E, so you will have to supplement this nutrient too. Pumpkin and sunflower seeds are also excellent sources. Taking large amounts of zinc (30mg a day or more) can inadvertently cause a copper deficiency, so if you plan to step up your intake of one, increase the other too.

There are now lots of multinutrient supplements formulated specifically for men, and the one herb they will all include is Saw palmetto. As well as being a natural anti-inflammatory, the active ingredient helps inhibit the action of an enzyme called 5-alpha-reductase which converts testosterone to its more active form, dihydrotestosterone (DHT). Saw palmetto also prevents DHT from binding in the prostate. In Europe, a number of studies have shown that taking 160mg of Saw palmetto extract, twice daily, is as effective as the prescription drug finasteride (Proscar), without the unwanted side effects.

Echinacea, burdock and the blue-green algae, all of which you can buy in liquid and tincture forms, can help keep the prostate healthy. If you are partial to herbal teas, one made from juniper berries has been shown to help dissolve unwanted sediment in the prostate, in the same way it can banish kidney stones. New research also suggests that the root of the much underrated nettle plant, when taken as a tea, can help reduce an enlarged prostate.

Diet plays an important role in prostate health, too. Increasing the amount of soya in the diet will provide higher levels of a powerful phytochemical called genistein, which researchers now believe can not only help prevent the development of a tumour, but also slow down the growth rate of an existing one. If you suffer from an inflamed prostate and if you are over the age of 40, and therefore more at risk than a younger man, it is a good idea to cut back on your red meat consumption and to cut out caffeine and tobacco. Try and drink six to eight glasses of clean water daily, but most of all cut down on animal fats. These contain oestrogens (female hormones used to fatten animals before slaughter), which stay in the meat. They are now known to lower testosterone levels and stimulate cell growth in the reproductive areas. In one study of 51,000 American men aged between 40 and 75, researchers were left in no doubt that prostate cancer was directly linked with the consumption of red meat.

PC-Spes is a new Chinese herbal remedy which even doctors are raving about. It was shown in clinical trials to shrink prostate cancer tumours in 87% of advanced cases where all other therapies had failed. It enhances the action of conventional treatments – chemotherapy and radiation – and lowers levels of a protein called Prostate Specific Antigen (PSA), which is an early marker for prostate cancer.

Psoriasis

Most common on the knees, scalp, legs and torso, the constant flaking, itching and scaling of the affected areas which characterise this condition (which affects 1% of the population) is the result of skin cells that have gone into over-drive, reproducing a thousand times faster than normal.

The rate at which cells divide is controlled by a complex balance between two compounds: cyclic adenosine monophosphate (AMP) and cyclic guanidine monophosphate (GMP). Higher than normal levels of GMP cause cells to divide too fast. Higher levels of AMP reduce the rate of cell replication. Oddly, studies have shown that a drop in the levels of both causes cells to rev up and divide too fast, again suggesting that the key to normal replication must be the balance between the two.

While stress, junk diets, bacteria, viruses, digestive disorders, liver and kidney problems, prescription drugs and multiple nutritional deficiencies have all been cited as the underlying cause, nobody has yet proven what really is to blame.

In 50% of cases there is a family history of the problem, and while conventional treatments may relieve the symptoms they do not tackle the root cause, which in some sufferers, for example, has been shown to be an intolerance to gluten.

One theory that is worth exploring is that this condition is linked with the body's inability to metabolise fatty acids. This can be easily remedied if you get into the habit of taking digestive enzymes (available in capsule form). Take one with each meal and another two capsules between times. Avoid citrus fruits, fried foods, wheat, white flour, dairy products and sugar. Step up the amount of vegetables, both raw and cooked, in your diet and take a tablespoon of olive oil daily with salad. Linseed or flaxseed oil is an excellent source of the fatty acids, so are the oily fish, especially mackerel and salmon.

Try to drink eight glasses of pure water each day, and get into the habit of juicing. Two large glasses of carrot and celery juice, each day, will help. Carrot, of course, is rich in vitamin A, which is crucial for skin health. Low levels have been found in psoriasis sufferers. Celery contains compounds called psoralens, which some researchers now believe may also help prevent psoriasis. These are also found in limes, lettuce, parsley, parsnips and lemons.

Avoid alcohol, which will only make your condition worse, and get into the habit of drinking organic nettle tea, which acts as a gentle liver detoxifying agent. Also, avoid rapid weight gain, which can also exacerbate the problem. A detoxification programme (see DeTox Diet, page 130) will decongest the colon and can help maintain normal weight.

Vitamin D (which is not a vitamin at all, but a hormone, see Chapter 4 on sunlight) plays a crucial role in cell replication. The best natural source is sunlight which may explain why psoriasis improves with exposure to the sun. Sunlight activates the pineal gland to regulate the hormones that act as chemical messengers and control all the body's natural functions.

Malformed cells, such as those that typify psoriasis, do not reach maturity before they slough off. According to holistic skin therapists, this could be because they are not producing enough solitrol – a hormone that is normally released through the skin. The best place to remedy this is at the Dead Sea in Israel or Jordan. It is the lowest point on earth, with an atmospheric haze that offers greater protection from the more harmful rays of the sun than any other place on earth. You also get the heat without the humidity that would otherwise accelerate mineral loss.

One of the minerals that has been linked with helping improve psoriasis is selenium, which is found in onions, garlic, chicken, seafood, tomatoes and broccoli. It is especially effective against psoriasis affecting the scalp. Few people get enough of it in their diet and so need to supplement with between 100–200mcg per day. Avoid stress-related outbreaks by taking a daily vitamin B complex.

Retinitas Pigmentosa

Retinitas pigmentosa (RP) is a rare inherited disorder (said to affect 1 in every 3,700 people) in which the retina – the light-sensitive membrane on the inner surface of the back of the eye – slowly and progressively degenerates, eventually causing blindness. The verdict with orthodox medicine is that there is no treatment and nothing you can do to stop this degeneration. Complementary medicine says otherwise.

Dr Eliot Berson, professor of Ophthalmology at Harvard Medical School, believes high doses of vitamin A can slow the loss of remaining eyesight by about 20% a year. He has been investigating the influence of vitamin A on the retina for 12 years, and has extensive research, including papers in the *American Journal of Clinical Nutrition*, which show that the high doses he recommends are entirely safe. He is adamant that retinitas pigmentosa is treatable and that if you take 15,000 iu (international units) of vitamin A per day, you can prolong your eyesight for up to 10 years, as long as you are not taking vitamin E simultaneously – which, he says, works adversely to lower the amount of A in the body.

Natural sources of pure vitamin A include liver and milk (if you eat carrots the vitamin A, in the form of carotene, will not be used by the eye), but for this condition you will not get a high enough dose from diet alone. Berson, who developed his theory after studying patient questionnaires which showed that those RP sufferers who were taking vitamin A in high doses preserved their vision for longer, says: 'My research shows the treatment for this condition is painfully simple, effective and safe.'

The simplest solution is to take Betacarotene which the liver then converts to vitamin A. Remember, this nutrient can be toxic in too high doses.

Raynaud's Syndrome/Poor Circulation

The circulatory system, comprising the heart, blood vessels and blood, is like the body's internal transport system, taking messages and materials, including nutrients, from one part to another. It also plays a key role in maintaining the internal balance of all your physical functions – a process known as homeostatis. It controls nutrient levels, waste disposal and the regulation of water and temperature.

With poor circulation, the efficiency of blood flow in the tiny capillaries – which are only five-thousandths of a millimetre in diameter and which ensure the exchange of materials between the blood and body tissues – is affected. Even the slightest drop in temperature can narrow the vessels, causing a condition known as Raynaud's Syndrome.

Raynaud's affects 9 times more women than men, and there are now an estimated 10 million sufferers in the UK alone. Yet when Anne Mawdsley, founder of the Raynaud's & Scleroderma Association was first diagnosed with it in 1975, she was told she had a rare condition which nobody knew much about.

The usual treatment for Raynaud's is prescription drugs which dilate the blood vessels. Unfortunately these drugs cannot target only those vessels affected, and so can cause problems such as headaches by dilating vessels in the brain, and nausea by affecting those in the stomach.

A more natural alternative is the circulation-boosting Chinese herb, Ginkgo biloba. In one recent, survey of Raynaud's sufferers testing a new product which combined the herb with phytosome (a natural plant chemical said to boost the absorption of the Ginkgo into the bloodstream), more than 70% said the supplement warmed their body and provided significant relief. Scientific researchers were so impressed, the first proper clinical trials are now under way.

Evening primrose oil has also performed well in clinical trials. In a double-blind study, 21 sufferers found that, compared with a placebo, the number of attacks and their severity decreased, although blood flow did not increase. These patients were taking between 3,000 and 6,000mg of evening primrose oil per day.

Ginger is a staple of Ayurvedic medicine, where it is used to warm the body and stimulate all the tissues, including the blood vessels. Start your day by adding a slice of fresh ginger root to honey, lemon and hot water to make a warming drink, or by adding fresh ginger to warmed fruit juice.

Lifestyle changes are important, too. Nicotine reduces blood flow to the extremities: so if you are a sufferer, stop smoking. The contraceptive pill can also affect circulation. Find alternatives if you suffer from Raynaud's.

Rhinitis

Traditional Chinese Medicine argues that the nose and the lungs are closely related, and that the lungs and the large intestine are like husband and wife. In acupuncture, for example, there is a connecting point between these organs. What this means is that an overload of toxicity from the intestines can overburden the lungs. The first thing most nutritionists will investigate when a client presents with this kind of allergy is that perennial bad guy of ill health – a yeast problem. Yeast toxins affect many organs in the body, and the symptoms can include nasal itching and rhinitis.

If you have taken antibiotics on a regular basis, if you eat a lot of chicken and red meat (these animals are pumped with antibiotics to promote more rapid growth, and the chemicals remain in the flesh after slaughter), if you have low energy levels and if you constantly feel bloated, you should suspect a yeast infection.

Hormonal disturbances, thanks to the contraceptive pill or Hormone Replacement Therapy (HRT), will also exacerbate the problem, as may some dairy products, which can disrupt the microflora of the intestine. Cut out dairy, yeast, sugar and meat (unless you buy organic meat) from your diet and see if your condition improves. There are many excellent books devoted to the problem of yeast infections (see Bibliography).

Rosacea

If you suffer from Rosacea – an alarming skin condition now believed to affect one adult in 15 – you are in serious danger of getting an inferiority complex. It is bad enough that this is a problem of mature skin that is hard to hide; what's worse is that it hardly merits a mention in most health manuals, alternative or otherwise. It is as if this troublesome condition does not even exist, except as a poor relation to acne.

Rosacea, pronounced *rose-ay-shah* is, in effect, an inflammatory skin disorder. The most common symptoms include facial redness across the nose, cheeks, chin and forehead, visibly damaged facial blood vessels and small, red inflammatory papules and pustules. It is not, though, the same as acne. Rosacea, for example, rarely causes blackheads, and most of the regimens recommended for acne are way too harsh for the supersensitive rosacea skin.

Most common among middle-aged women, the problem may start innocently enough. The first sign, for example, is often a temporary flushing of the face, especially after a hot drink, spicy food or when you walk into an overheated room. In men it can cause the kind of bulbous swelling of the nose that we usually associate with alcoholism. It can flare up for no obvious reason, and while one theory is that it is caused by an underlying disorder of the blood vessels supplying the face, nobody knows for sure. Some sufferers have a permanently ruddy or florid complexion. For others, it may not ever look that bad but the affected skin often stings badly.

I have heard Rosacea sufferers describe how they have visited the doctor for a different complaint and walked in and out of the surgery with nobody mentioning the chronic skin condition that has so blatantly stamped its mark all over their face. No wonder, then, that so many sufferers hide at home, waiting patiently for a flare-up to pass.

Doctors are generally too busy to swot up on unsexy subjects like chronic skin inflammation, and rarely have a better suggestion than telling patients they will have to learn to live with it. This is just not true. There are things you can do to manage and even alleviate the symptoms, but these changes will take longer to have an effect than low-dose Roaccutane, which is the conventional solution. This last-resort retinoid cream will clear the problem – but usually only for as long as you keep taking it. And it can come with some pretty unpleasant side-effects including a dry mouth and depression. Also, once you stop taking it your Rosacea will come back.

According to Helen Sher, the Canadian skin specialist who runs a now world-famous clinic treating all skin disorders, but mainly acne and Rosacea, the key to her treatment programme is water. She says it is crucial to remoisturise the skin by splashing your face with body-temperature water twice a day, when you get up and before you go to bed. The Sher Skincare system is a range of products for sensitive acne and Rosacea skins. It is expensive and will not work for everyone, but thousands of Rosacea sufferers around the world swear by it.

According to skin experts, there is no question that Rosacea is linked to digestion and affected by stress. Environmental factors, such as sudden exposure to sunlight, wind or temperature changes, will make the condition worse, as will red wine and caffeine drinks.

For gut healing and a general detoxification of the digestive tract, complementary health practitioners recommend taking an amino acid called L-glutamine – but you must avoid this if you are pregnant or have kidney or liver problems. Vitamin A plays a role in the formation of new skin, and supplements of zinc will help prevent skin scarring. Vitamin C with bioflavanoids has been shown to strengthen capillaries as well as immune function, and iodine-rich kelp can provide missing minerals that maintain good skin tone.

The range of food triggers reported by Rosacea sufferers is vast – liver, yeast, red plums, steak, chocolate, cheese, spinach, figs and citrus fruits to name but a few. To find out which foods exacerbate your own problem, you need to adopt an elimination diet where you cut out the suspected food for several weeks and then re-introduce it to see if symptoms flare up again. Keeping a food diary will make this task easier.

Dr Geoffrey Nase is a Rosacea sufferer who has spent five years investigating natural treatments for his condition. His current recommendations are to take a form of vitamin C called Ester C, along with grape seed extract. This combination, he says, has excellent anti-inflammatory properties, strengthens the blood vessel walls and decreases swelling of the affected areas. He suggests, if you weigh under 10 stone 10 (150lb), you work up to 1,000mg of Ester C and 200mg of grape seed extract, three times a day. For those over this weight, aim for 2,000mg of Ester C and 200mg of grape seed extract. Be warned, though, building up to these high doses of vitamin C can cause temporary diarrhoea.

Acupuncture (see Hands-on, page 261) can also be helpful and is worth investigating. There is lots of anecdotal evidence for its efficacy with skin problems, but little in the way of hard science. What has been suggested is that during treatment, among the chemicals released by the pituitary gland, is a natural steroid called adrenocorticotrophic hormone. If this is true, then it is holistic healing at its finest, since it is a treatment that is triggering true healing from the inside out.

Sarcoidosis

This is a disease which tends to develop in young adults. It happens when abnormal collections of inflammatory cells called *granulomas* form in the body's different organs, especially the lungs. Some doctors believe it is the legacy of an infection, others suggest it is an abnormal immune system response. Many sufferers have no symptoms at all, and the problem is only discovered by accident when it shows up on a chest X-ray taken for other reasons. Fever, weight loss and aching joints are all likely symptoms. It is seldom fatal and usually burns itself out within two years. In fact, more than two-thirds of those with lung sarcoidosis, for example, will have no symptoms at all after nine years.

The conventional treatment is steroids, but these come with side-effects and so many holistic practitioners prefer to try and tackle the possible underlying causes. One theory, for example, is that this is an auto-immune condition caused by an accumulation of acidifying protein residues in the connective tissues.

The way to avoid this is by controlling the amount of protein in the diet to avoid any build-up between meals. This special diet was first reported in

The Proceedings of the Royal Society of Medicine in 1937 after it was shown to help a dozen bed-bound arthritic patients get up and moving again, but it was never taken up by orthodox practitioners. Instead, it was left to the holistic healers, among them Benedict Lust, one of the founding fathers of naturopathy, who promoted it widely. As well as arthritis, this special method of Dietary Cleansing (see page 135) has also been shown to help treat migraines and muscular rheumatism.

A cleansing programme of eating, rather than a diet plan, it is safe to administer yourself and is enhanced by taking herbal remedies such as echinacea, Siberian ginseng and aloe vera, which can all help normalise immune function. If you feel nervous about embarking on one, see a qualified health practitioner.

Please note that you should avoid vitamin D supplementation if you have this condition.

Scars

You may want to invest in a sharp needle because, with many natural treatments, it is what is *inside* the vitamin or essential oil capsules that can help accelerate the healing of scar tissue. Many practitioners use vitamin E massaged onto the affected site once the wound has healed, but wheatgerm oil is just as good and will help the redness fade completely even when the scarring is severe.

The world's best holistic skin therapists also use an oil that was originally developed as an anti-wrinkle lotion. *Rosa mosqueta* (rose hip) oil should also be massaged onto the scar tissue once the wound has healed.

In the Ayurvedic tradition, doctors mix a little sandalwood oil with a little aloe vera cream to help reduce scarring. Throughout India, sandalwood, which is said to regenerate tissue, is used to treat a wide range of skin problems.

Aloe vera is very helpful in the treatment of all wounds and is now used in many skin preparations. A more unappealing remedy in the West is castor oil. It may sound horrid but, according to herbalists, it can be used to 'draw out' toxic accumulations, such as cysts, tumours and warts, and its emollient effect means it will help soften and erradicate scars. (For suppliers of these oils, see Resources.)

You might also like to investigate a treatment that is new to the UK but which was developed in Russia, where it was first used to fine-tune the bodies of their astronauts. KOSMED – the name is short for cosmic medicine device – has just been approved officially for pain relief in Britain and so far, this is the only claim those who know how to use it are making. That said, I have heard strong anecdotal evidence that it can also help heal scars. The device looks like a TV remote control and works by triggering the body's own healing powers to complete the job of healing at the affected site (see KOSMED Healing, page 297).

Sex Drive

I get lots of letters from both men and women asking how they can spice up a flagging libido. The easy answer is with a herb called yohimbe – a supplement that is so hot, supplies practically walk off the shelves in America where it is sold over the counter. Extracted from the bark of a West African tree, yohimbe has long been used as a folk remedy for impotence and as an aphrodisiac, and while there are no scientific studies to support such claims for it, plenty of people swear to its potency in bed. It would, I have no doubt, sell equally well outside the States, but in the UK it is not licensed for sale, which means we have to find an alternative.

Asparagus and artichokes are both said to be good aphrodisiacs – but there are only so many asparagus tips a girl can eat, and only a very few men who will find the sight of butter dripping down her chin remotely appealing.

Damiana (*Turnera diffusa*) which is said to help impotence, relieve anxiety, promote well-being and act as a sexual stimulant for both sexes, is probably a better option. Traditionally used as an aphrodisiac for men and women in Central America, it helps rebalance hormones and has mildly stimulating properties, said to enhance feelings of alertness and energy. One theory is that it slightly irritates the urethra in men, thus sensitising the penis and making it more responsive to stimulation.

Damiana is also an effective natural laxative, so if your herbalist has prescribed it for constipation there is no need to sack him or her just yet. For sexual performance, take it in tincture form for a quick hit. Mix 10–30 drops of tincture in fruit juice and take it half an hour before meals.

Agnus castus is another herb that can help boost your sex life. Frequently prescribed to rebalance the hormones in menopausal and pre-menstrual women, many people are surprised to learn it can work just as effectively in men. It reduces levels of prolactin in the body, which controls milk production in women and which tends to be too high in cases of low thyroid function. Vitamin B_6 can do a similar job; it is found in foods such as cabbage, molasses, oatmeal, chicken and milk.

Some simple dietary exclusions can also help a flagging libido, especially for men. Eliminating wheat, beer, milk, cheese and alcohol can help prevent bloating and constipation, both conditions that can affect your interest in sex. A deficiency in zinc, which again is common in both sexes, can also adversely affect sexual appetite. White flecks on the fingernails are a sign of this deficiency, which can easily be remedied by taking a zinc supplement to provide 25mg a day.

If you spend a lot of time in front of a computer or the television, then your sex life could be adversely affected by the pulsed electromagnetic radiations (PEMR) which have now been linked with reduced fertility and libido and increased tiredness. In one study, for example, human testicle cells exposed to radiation from a computer screen for 24 hours had a 300% increase in mortality, compared with unexposed cells. There is a massive European study into these effects underway, but if this is an area that already concerns you, you could investigate the protective benefits of one of the popular pendant-style EMR-Bioshield devices.

If you just want to set a more romantic mood for love, there are plenty of essential oils to choose from. Try ylang ylang, which is traditionally used to promote love and sex, or jasmine, which promotes love, sex and sleep (as if most men need any help with sleep!), and which is known as the King of Essential Oils.

Shingles

Shingles (or herpes zoster) is an infection that produces a very painful eruption of fluid-filled blisters. It is caused by the same virus responsible for chickenpox. It enters the cranial or spinal nerves, where it stays latent until activated by a minor infection, local trauma, stress, nutritional deficiencies, food intolerances or exposure to sunlight. The symptoms, which signal an outbreak, usually include a stinging area of skin, chills, fever, nausea, diarrhoea or problems with urination, followed a few days later by an outbreak of fluid-filled blisters. And, while most of us think of this as an older person's disease, it is increasingly affecting younger adults.

Antiviral drugs may be given to shorten the duration of the skin eruption (and aspirin or codeine may be prescribed for the temporary relief of pain in adults), but there is no drug that can eliminate the virus itself. What you can do, though, is accelerate your recovery from an attack by adopting a diet that is rich in live yoghurt, oily fish, organic fruits, vegetables, nuts and seeds. These are all high in antioxidants, which will boost the immune system. It is also important to drink plenty of fluids – especially teas brewed from herbs such as Echinacea, golden seal and dandelion, which also support the immune system.

Nutritional consultants will also recommend bromelain, an enzyme found naturally in pineapples, which, in doses of 250mg three times a day, has been shown to be as effective as the orthodox medicine Zovirax in enhancing immune function and tackling the herpes virus.

There are also excellent homeopathic remedies for shingles – including Rhus tox which is usually given when the patient complains of itchy, painful blisters. If you are serious about homeopathy and your condition is a recurring one, I recommend you have a constitutional diagnosis with a qualified practitioner, who will tailor-make a remedy for you (see page 76).

Applying vitamin E to the skin can help relieve pain and reduce scarring. So can Cider Vinegar. During an outbreak, avoid eating and using citrus fruits including orange, grapefruit, lemon and lime.

A weakened immune system is the primary cause of shingles; see page 166.

Sinusitis

Chronic sinusitis (that is, repeated infections) is frequently associated with an allergic response either to food or the environment. Symptoms can include nasal congestion and discharge, fever, chills and headaches, pain, tenderness, redness and swelling over the affected area. When the condition is chronic you may also suffer with a non-productive cough. In a small number of cases there is an underlying dental infection, but any factor which causes swelling and fluid retention of the mucous membranes of the sinuses can block drainage and result in inflamation and even infection.

Alcohol, dust, pollen, hot spicy foods and even petrol fumes can all exacerbate the problem, so try and eliminate these from your life. Cut down on the amount of wheat, dairy, eggs and citrus foods in your diet, and try to eliminate caffeine and refined sugars.

You will also need to boost your immune system. A good start is to take at least 500mg of vitamin C, twice a day. Also, take a good general multivitamin supplement and zinc lozenges (15mg daily). Bromelain, an enzyme derived from pineapple juice, has powerful anti-inflammatory properties and will also enhance the absorption of the other nutrients and supplements you are taking. In the throes of an infection, take up to three 500mg tablets daily.

You should try to get plenty of rest and drink large amounts of fluids in the form of diluted vegetable juices and herbal teas. One of the most effective herbal remedies for sinus infections is golden seal (*Hydrastis canadensis*), which you can take either as a tea or in tincture form. When you are congested, a cold flannel laid across the bridge of the nose will also bring relief.

Smoking

The key to stopping smoking is not to give up when each attempt to quit fails (each time you stop, it will be for longer), and to get all the help you can. You will also do yourself a big favour if you avoid other smokers and places where people do smoke until you are sure you really have beaten an addiction which many doctors believe to be just as powerful and insidious as heroin. It took me four years to stop smoking completely. I used a combination of willpower, nicotine patches, avoidance therapy (steering clear of friends who still smoked) and drinking endless cups of peppermint tea, which I would make each time I wanted a cigarette.

The homeopathic remedy most often recommended to help those who want to stop smoking is Caladium 6c, which comes from the American *Arum* plant and which has been shown to help alleviate tobacco cravings. A herb called *Avena sativa* – which you will know better by its common name of oats – will also help by supporting the nervous system as you withdraw from your regular intake of nicotine. The best way to benefit from this is to drink organic oat juice (available in health stores). You also need to eat a diet that is high in fruit and vegetables. This helps beat cravings by changing the pH of the body, making it less acidic (cigarettes make it more acidic).

It takes three months for all traces of nicotine to leave your system. After that, any cravings you suffer are psychological. It helps to know this, because when this deadline has gone and you still feel you must smoke, you'll know it is your mind playing tricks and that the craving will pass. There are lots of herbal formulations which will help. Napiers, for example, make one called Aim Calm which contains valerian, vervain, skullcap and hops and does just what the name implies. (Please note that you should not take Aim Calm if you are pregnant or depressed.) Lobelia is also an effective tool in the battle to stop smoking. It stops cravings by attaching to the same receptor sites as nicotine and helps restore clean lungs. Large doses can cause nausea, so herbalists suggest you take it in the form of a cough syrup.

Sperm Problems (Low Sperm Count)

It takes three months to form a mature sperm and researchers believe it is during this developmental stage that the sperm is most at risk from environmental toxins. Sperm count in the West has slumped by 50% in the last five decades, and I can't understand why more men are not more frightened by this. One theory, now backed by the Medical Research Council, is that substances called xeno-oestrogens produced by chemicals used in the environment are responsible. To minimise contact with these, adopt a diet that is rich in organic fruits and vegetables and cut down on using plastics to store foods. (Keep leftovers in a glass bowl, and stop using cling film.)

The first priority in protecting mature sperm is to avoid over-heating the testicles. Men with a low sperm count should not take hot baths or wear tight underclothing, both of which can affect the motility of the sperm. Alcohol and smoking adversely affect sperm, so cut both of these out too. Scientists have now found a higher risk of childhood cancers in children born to fathers who smoke during pregnancy, even when the mother was a non-smoker. They believe toxins from cigarettes can damage the sperm's DNA, so it is really important that men, as well as women, who want to conceive, should give up cigarettes.

Zinc is the single most important nutrient in a man's reproductive system. Zinc citrate (between 15–30mg a day) has been shown to help boost sperm count. Vitamin E and selenium are both important antioxidants, which will further help prevent cell damage caused by toxins. Several amino acids, which are the building blocks of protein, are also crucial to the formation of healthy sperm. L-arginine and L-taurine are probably the most important; you can buy these in supplement form too.

Spots

You may think you eat a healthy diet, but you need to keep a careful eye on the amount of saturated fats you are eating as they can exacerbate skin problems. Use cold-pressed vegetable oils, for example, but don't cook with them because the heat causes a chemical change of the healthier polyunsaturated fats, leading to something called trans fats. Ironically, these are as unhealthy as the saturated fats you were trying to avoid in the first place.

Iodine may aggravate skin complaints, so cut out iodized table salt and make sure you are taking a good multivitamin with vitamins A and B complex, plus zinc and selenium, all of which promote healthy skin.

A homemade herbal poultice (see page 75) of grated cucumber, cooked and puréed organic carrots plus oatmeal cooked in water will also deep-cleanse the skin. Apply and leave this on your face for half an hour and then wash off with cold water.

Instead of using a chemical commercial cleanser, keep your skin spot-free by cleaning it with equal parts of lemon juice and purified water. At night, take a tip from the Ayurvedic practitioners and massage equal parts of sesame, sunflower, flax seed, almond and olive oils sparingly into the skin.

To bring out lesions, steam the face over hot water mixed with 10 drops of tea tree oil, then dab the spots with marigold tincture or a cube of ice.

Poor digestion and elimination is often the root cause of bad skin or periodic outbreaks of spots. Detoxify by changing your diet or by taking dandelion or burdock in tincture form. Dissolve the herb of your choice in warm water and take three times a day.

You can also help bring a spot to a head – and prevent reinfection – using tea tree oil, but make sure you buy a product which supplies enough of the active ingredient to be effective. For this problem I recommend the excellent Dessert Essence brand (for suppliers, see Resources). For information about treating boils, which may be a sign of diabetes, see page 103.

Surgery

If you are having an operation, you know your body is going to suffer tissue damage and serious bruising. This is, of course, an opportunity to use complementary medicine in the truest sense of the word.

Once in hospital you are in the one place where you are more likely to get an infection than anywhere else – one of my all-time favourite quotes is that from a member of the British Medical Association's (BMA) occupational health committee, Dr Joe Kearns, who was once head of health and safety for a big food manufacturer. He told a BMA annual conference that hospital patients have less protection against infection than a pork pie on a production line: 'On a ward of patients with open wounds, the consultant and his team will wander from one to the next without washing their hands,' he warned.

As well as your psyche, when you go into hospital, your liver, digestion and immune system are also going to take a serious battering from the anaesthetic and painkilling drugs which are routinely prescribed. So, if ever there was a time to take some responsibility for your own health and well-being, the run-up to surgery is it.

Although, as general rule, I strongly recommend you see a qualified homoeopath who can make a constitutional diagnosis (see page 76) to find the right remedy for you, I also always point people in the direction of homoeopathy before they go into hospital. Homoeopathy is safe and will not interfere with your other medications. It is also very specific, so you should be able to figure, from the type of surgery you will have and your likely reaction to the ordeal, which remedy will suit you.

I often get letters from people asking if the same remedies are necessary when they are having surgery for cosmetic reasons. The answer, of course, is that while you might know this surgery is voluntary, to your body the trauma is the same.

There are three main steps to preparing for an operation. First you need to protect yourself from infection. You need to minimise the shock of the operation to your body, and you will want to know how you can reduce the lividity of the inevitable scarring you will be left with.

Make sure you are in as good a shape as possible before your operation by boosting your immune system (see page 166). Of the many ways to do this, taking the herb echinacea is the simplest. Take 20 drops in water or juice, three or four times a day, starting 14 days before the date of your operation.

A week before surgery, start taking 15,000 iu (international units) of vitamin A daily. This powerful antioxidant will help your immune system fight the threat of infection and will accelerate wound-healing. Step this dose up to 50,000 iu for two days before and two days after surgery, unless you are pregnant, in which case do not exceed 15,000 iu.

Also, two days before going to hospital you should begin a course of high-potency homoeopathic Arnica, which will lessen the bruising, swelling and soreness. Take four pillules of 30c Arnica at night and in the morning, and again just before surgery. Remember to tip these from the container directly under the tongue, to avoid touching them (which can destroy the remedy's activity).

Despite improvements in modern anaesthetics, 25% of the population still react badly after surgery. As one of these, I can vouch for the efficacy of another homoeopathic remedy – Nux vomica. The name says it all and, again, take a high-potency 30c strength.

The onslaught of prescription drugs will take its toll on your poor liver. Support it, before the operation, by taking the herb milk thistle. The active ingredient is silymarin, which has been shown to help regenerate liver cells. Take as directed on the bottle, between meals, three times a day, for a week before surgery and two weeks after.

Lots of people now know that rubbing vitamin E oil onto a scar can help speed up the healing process (to do this, break open a standard soft capsule), but not many have discovered the fantastic regenerating properties of the simple rosehip. This tip was passed to me by the holistic skin therapist Jane Waters, and people have been writing to me ever since I passed it on to say how thrilled they are with the results. *Rosa mosqueta* is sourced from the Brazilian rainforest and was originally developed to help reduce wrinkles around the eyes. To minimise scarring, apply to the wound once it has healed, massaging it into the affected area.

Certain foods will also help your body prepare for the shock of surgery, especially those that are rich in an amino acid called L-arginine. This stimulates the thymus gland, which in turn stores the infection-fighting T-lymphocytes or T-cells until they are needed to ward off disease. Ironically, levels of L-arginine drop during times of stress, but you can increase them again by eating more poultry and fish, which are excellent natural sources, and by taking a supplement.

I once had the misfortune to be bed-ridden on a hospital ward for two months, so I know all the pitfalls. If the stodgy unappetising food doesn't finish you off, the antibiotic-resistant infections that are becoming more prevalent might. Protect your digestion and your general health by making sure you are scrupulous about personal hygiene. Drink 2 litres of pure, still water a day to flush toxins out of your body; soothe the lining of the gut, which will be disturbed by antibiotics, by drinking aloe vera juice. Try and keep to as healthy a diet as you can, and count the days until they let you out again! Call me biased, but I left hospital twice as sick as I was when I first went it. It took two years to struggle back to good health, and I have not been near a doctor or a surgeon since.

Teeth

Companies which make chemical-free toothpastes have re-discovered a sweet herb called Stevia which, according to clinical trials, may help prevent tooth decay (sadly, at the time of going to press, this herb had been unexpectedly withdrawn from over-the-counter sales in the UK). Charlotte Vontz, a former chemist and the founder of the UK's Green People Company, warns that the gums absorb 90% of what you put on them, and says there is evidence that sodium lauryl sulphate – a foaming agent used in most toothpastes – has been shown, in high concentrations, to dissolve protein in the body and so may actually make gums weaker.

For mild toothache, fresh figs rubbed onto the gums can help soothe the pain thanks to their anti-inflammatory properties. They are a good alternative to the bitter taste of clove oil, which is more commonly used. Prickly ash is known in folk medicine as the 'toothache tree' because its bark was chewed for relief – but for really good dental health, take a tip from the rabbits and chew on carrots. They contain a large amount of silicon, which not only strengthens the connective tissue in the jaw but also boosts the absorption of calcium. This is a great help in strengthening the teeth of younger children, for whom chewing on carrot sticks can encourage the development of the lower jaw and prevent overcrowding of the teeth.

The practice of bleaching to whiten teeth has now been discontinued in the UK, leaving people even more dependent on whitening toothpastes. Of these, a brand called Janina promises to wipe the floor with most competitors. In early trials at the Royal London Dental School, patients who used Janina for six months developed healthier gums, whiter teeth and fresher breath than those using other makes. The reason, according to Dr Edward Lynch (who carried out the trials) is that while most toothpastes contain just three ingredients to fight plaque, tartar and gingivitis, Janina boasts 16. It does, though, contain sodium lauryl sulphate, which you may prefer to avoid.

Thread Veins

Vitamin K cream is commonly prescribed to help fade away thread veins, broken capillaries and bruises. It can speed up the healing process in sun-damaged skin and is frequently used to prevent scarring after cosmetic procedures such as laser resurfacing. There is scant clinical evidence to show how it works, but anecdotally, many people swear by it.

The product I recommend you try is Vitamin K Creme Plus by Jason Natural Cosmetics, a company which has specialised in the development of therapeutic treatments for a range of skin conditions for more than 40 years. This cream contain 3% vitamin K, plus 30 additional natural ingredients, including the powerful antioxidant Gingko biloba to improve circulation and the immune booster grapefruit seed extract (see Resources for suppliers).

Recommended for toning down skin redness, minimising the appearance of broken blood vessels and bruising and for treating varicose veins, this cream is also formulated with calendula (from the marigold plant), which helps normalise skin structure.

Bilberry, more commonly used to maintain good eyesight, can also strengthen blood vessels and help prevent thread veins and in Europe, clinical trials using active ingredients taken from the horse chestnut (conker) tree have proved to be as effective as any conventional remedy.

Thyroid Health

An over-active thyroid is more common in women than men, and may affect up to 2% of the adult female population – the most common cause is Graves disease, which is an autoimmune disorder.

The thyroid gland produces hormones which regulate growth, maturation and the body's metabolism. An over-active thyroid produces too much hormone, the symptoms of which can include insomnia, disturbed bowel movements, increased appetite accompanied by weight loss, high blood pressure, nervousness and a faster heartbeat. The main complaint of those suffering from an under-active thyroid is exhaustion.

Since the thyroid controls energy production, the metabolism of sugars and fats, your growth rate, the conversion of vitamin A into betacarotene, your heart rate, your blood pressure, your rate of breathing, mental alertness and the libido, it is no wonder, when it malfunctions, that you feel so very low.

Even if sufferers eventually opt for surgery, there are many lifestyle and nutritional changes which help support normal thyroid function. These include reducing stress, cutting out stimulants such as cigarettes, coffee and sugary foods, eating small, frequent meals, and taking a supplement of B vitamins, especially B_{12}.

Foods which help to moderate excessive thyroid activity include members of the brassica family such as brussels sprouts, cabbage, cauliflower, broccoli, kale and turnip. It is important to support metabolic functioning with a good multivitamin. Check there is no deficiency in zinc or magnesium, and make sure your diet is rich in fatty acids (abundant in, for example, oily fish).

To support an under-active thyroid, you will need to boost your dietary intake of iodine. Eat more sea vegetables, especially kelp and dulse, and switch to iodised salt. Again, make sure your intake remains moderate – in excess, these foods will have the opposite effect.

To be effective in the body, iodine needs the presence of an amino acid called tyrosine, and this, in turn, needs enough vitamins E, A, B_2, B_3, B_6 and C, as well as copper, zinc and selenium. Organic foods contain up to four times more selenium than non-organic, so it would be worth making the changeover if you haven't done so already.

An enlarged thyroid can be a sign of a congested liver. Milk thistle, which works to regenerate damaged liver cells, can help remedy this. Drinking organic nettle tea will also discourage further stagnation. The usual cause of a swollen and sluggish liver is a diet that is too high in rich and saturated fatty foods.

You can take iodine-rich sea vegetables in supplement form, but in the kitchen add kombu and kelp sea plants to beans as you cook them. The minerals in these sea nutrients help balance the protein and oils in the beans, making them more digestible. They also soften the tough fibres in beans and other foods they are cooked with.

Never stop medication for thyroid complaints without medical supervision.

Tinnitus

The ringing, hissing and buzzing in the ears which are typical of tinnitis make it highly disruptive for sufferers; while it may not be easy to determine the cause, there are many lifestyle factors which will exacerbate the condition. Loud noise, poor circulation, food sensitivities and stimulants such as caffeine and nicotine can all make it worse. Permanent, severe tinnitus is very hard to treat but changing your diet may help.

Some studies have shown patients who switch to a low-fat, low-cholesterol diet, for example, experience a significant reduction in symptoms. There is also some evidence that taking zinc supplementation may help, too (take 30mg for two months).

Ginkgo biloba, the Chinese herb which is used to boost circulation, has shown very promising results when used in the treatment of tinnitus. In one study of 33 sufferers, 12 patients recovered completely and five more showed marked improvement. If you take this route, be patient. It can take two weeks for the effect of Ginkgo biloba to kick in, and the longer you take it, the greater the benefits.

Travel Remedies

Tucking a gnarled rhizome of fresh ginger into your travel bag may cause some consternation when you pass through security at the airport, but you'll be glad you remembered it when, for example, you find yourself being bounced up and down in the back of the truck taking you to that remote Caribbean hillside retreat or when you've eaten a dodgy seafood paella.

Ginger – or Gian Jiang as it is known in Traditional Chinese Medicine – may not sound like the sexiest solution to travel sickness and nausea, but it has long been used to treat morning sickness in pregnant women and it really works. It contains a natural antibiotic, so as well as stimulating the circulation to warm up the body it is also effective against flu, cramps and stomach upsets. Of course you don't have to take the root form with you, but if you are putting together your own alternative travel kit, ginger oil or capsules should be included, and if you are travelling to a very cold climate you can make a tea from fresh ginger, which will warm your body from the inside out.

This is just one of many natural herbal and homeopathic travel remedies you can use to treat a range of minor ailments and conditions while travelling or on holiday. If you accidentally stay out too long and get burned by the sun, for example, echinacea cream will soothe and accelerate the rate at which the damaged skin heals. If it's insect bites you need to concern yourself with, dilute citronella, lavender, eucalyptus or tea tree oils in an almond oil base and apply to the skin.

You can pack a rather unusual remedy to treat jellyfish stings (see alternative travel kit checklist, below), and avoid the uncomfortable and sometimes embarrassing symptoms of irritable bowel syndrome (IBS) by travelling with psyllium seeds and remembering to eat live yoghurt, which will go some way to help keep the balance of the flora in your gut healthy despite a change in climate and diet.

For long-haul travellers, the one condition most likely to cost you at least one or two days of your holiday is jet lag. Again, complementary medicine can provide a solution. The most talked about product to counter the disorientating effects of a disturbed body clock is melatonin (see Insomnia, page 173). A hormone produced naturally by the pea-sized pineal gland in the brain, this is the chemical, which regulates your natural bodyclock. Levels peak at night, when you sleep, and drop off again during the day. While melatonin is only available on prescription in the UK (it is not licensed and so has not been authorised for sale by the Medicines Control Agency), you can still buy it freely over the counter in the US or via the Internet.

A less well-known but extremely effective anti-jet lag supplement is 5-HTP (5-hydroxytryptophan). Sometimes described as a natural alternative to antidepressants including Prozac, it works by enhancing the production of serotonin, a hormone produced in the brain which plays a role in mood, sleep and appetite and which is the precursor to melatonin. Low levels are linked with anxiety and sleep disorders, but while some antidepressants work by stopping the brain from using too much serotinin too quickly, 5-HTP actually boosts levels by increasing the amount of serotonin being produced.

Even if you don't pack an alternative travel kit, you can often treat common complaints with everyday items. Sometimes the bacteria causing severe diarrhoea, for example, can be eliminated just by drinking a cup of tea. This is no ordinary cup of tea, of course. The trick is to make it very strong (use four teabags or an equivalent amount of loose tea) so that the tannin, which is a natural antibacterial agent, will kill off the offending bug. If you have nothing else to treat sunburn, smother the affected area with cold yoghurt from the fridge, or add cucumber juice to a cold water compress to help cool the burning skin.

Alternative Travel Kit

Ginger: Stops nausea and travel sickness. Also eases cramps and stomach pains. The easiest way to take it is in tincture form. Take 1–2 drops directly under the tongue.

Aloe vera: Formulated specifically for sunburn, Aloe Max, for example, is a gel from New Zealand, which also contains chlorophyll, to help the skin repair after sun damage. For suppliers, see Resources.

Probiotics: Will help prevent and treat the dreaded Traveller's Tummy (see Immune System-Boosting, page 166). Stomach upsets – which are an occupational hazard when you are travelling – can disturb the natural balance of bacteria in the gut, allowing more pathogenic bugs to flourish. This imbalance can, in turn, cause IBS, candida, chronic fatigue, food allergies, rheumatoid arthritis and depression. If you buy capsules, make sure they have an enteric coating to protect the good bacteria as they pass through the acidic stomach to the more alkaline, less hostile gut.

Nettle tea: An excellent liver tonic, this simple brew will not only help your recovery when you overindulge, but is also effective against allergies such as hay fever. It can relieve inflammation caused by an allergic response and clear congestion in the nose and chest. Buy an organic brand.

5-Hydroxytryptophan (5-HTP): Beats jet lag by boosting levels of serotonin, the mood-controlling hormone produced in the brain which is a precursor to the manufacture of melatonin, the hormone which regulates the natural body clock. It won't work straight away, so start taking it two weeks before your departure date.

Goldenseal: One of the most potent antibacterial, antifungal and antiviral agents known to man, this herb can be combined with a probiotic treatment both to prevent and treat stomach upsets. Combine with echinacea to boost the immune system and ward off a cold. It can be expensive but it lasts a long time. Take just 20 drops, three times a day.

Echinacea cream: Accelerates wound-healing and is excellent for serious sunburn. The UK supplier Bioforce (see Resources) sells an echinacea cream, which also contains wild pansy to nourish damaged and traumatised skin. Avoid burning altogether with a lavender sunblock. Neal's Yard Remedies (see Resources) have a very effective block, which is recommended for those areas which burn more quickly.

Arnica 30c: If you take nothing else, make sure you pack this homoeopathic remedy. It can reduce bleeding, inflammation and bruising and is prescribed by homoeopaths to counter shock and promote rapid healing. It is also effective against jet lag.

Pyrogen 200c: Although homoeopathic remedies are more effective when based on a constitutional diagnosis by a qualified practitioner, for emergencies, self-prescribing is better than nothing. Pyrogen is useful in treating both food poisoning and fevers that are a result of flu, a septic infection or just rotten food. Typically, symptoms of these conditions will make you alternate between feeling cold and chilly and hot and sweaty, with palpitations.

Citronella, eucalyptus or lavender oils: Stop insects from biting in the first place. Essential oils should never be applied straight on to the skin. Dilute them first in an almond base oil. Dissolve 10–20 drops into an eggcup of the base oil. This way, you can mix different oils.

Ulcers

While stress may play a role in exacerbating stomach ulcers, it is not, contrary to what most people believe, usually the primary cause. Neither is spicy food. Thrusting corporate executives, for example, get ulcers at exactly the same rate as those with much less stress in their lives, which suggests there must be some other dominant factor at play.

This factor goes by the name of *Helicobacter pylori* (*H. pylori*) – a spiral-shaped bacteria that has been found to be present in 90% of patients with peptic ulcers. One of very few microorganisms to be resistant to the antibacterial properties of the stomach's strong acid secretions, *H. pylori* protects itself by producing a compound called urase which neutralises these acids. It is then free to burrow through the protective mucous membranes of stomach and duodenum (the upper area of the intestine, just below the stomach).

This infection, which causes both chronic irritation and inflammation, leaves many sufferers dependent on a constant diet of antacids to relieve the discomfort. The symptoms range from blunt, gnawing or sharp stomach pain to lower backache, discomfort when passing stools, headaches, choking sensations and itching. Bleeding occurs only when the ulcer has penetrated a blood vessel, a condition which then requires medical intervention.

There appears to be a genetic predisposition towards getting an ulcer, since large numbers of the population – an estimated 50% of all those over the age of 50 – carry *H. pylori* in the gut but not all those infected in this way go on to develop ulcers.

Eating certain foods can provide temporary relief, but again there are many fallacies around which ones soothe and which exacerbate the problem. Far from aggravating an ulcer, many spicy foods have now been found to have little or no effect on stomach ulcers or the lining of the stomach. Indeed, cayenne pepper has been shown in some studies to strengthen the stomach lining. Another mistake is to think that milk will coat the stomach lining and thus provide a measure of protection.

The foods and fluids you should avoid are those that stimulate the stomach's acid secretions. These include fatty foods, fruit juices, cola and other carbonated drinks, coffee (including decaffeinated), chocolate and alcohol. Eggs, fish, bread, starchy grains and sugary foods will also promote acid secretion.

A lot of nutritional advice is based on synergy – the notion that the foods we eat affect each other in the body. If you are trying to create a less acidic and more alkaline environment, you need to be eating more of the so-called alkaline foods which include potatoes, avocados, squash, cottage cheese and blue or purple grapes. Red and white beans and unpolished rice all mop up acid in the stomach, while chlorophyll-rich liquid algae will heal inflammation. Bananas, figs, antioxidant green tea and kale can all strengthen the stomach lining too.

Of all the foods that can help when you do have an ulcer, the humble cabbage is king. Not boiled or stir-fried, but juiced and swallowed down quickly while the live enzymes are still fresh. For both stomach and duodenal ulcers, drink one half-cupful of freshly juiced cabbage two or three times a day between meals. If you hate the colour and taste, flavour it with a little carrot juice.

Cabbage contains a less well-known nutrient called vitamin U and a substance called quercetin, which is also found in red onions. This is a bioflavanoid which not only has anti-inflammatory properties but which has been found to inhibit the growth of *H. pylori*. The recommended dose if you plan to take this in supplement form is 500mg, three times a day. Another bioflavanoid, called apigenin, is found in camomile – which explains why many ulcer sufferers find camomile herbal tea so soothing.

Liquorice root has long been used in traditional medicine to calm inflamed and injured mucous membranes in the digestive tract. It protects the area by increasing the production of mucin and is, again, a rich source of other bioflavanoids which can (according to laboratory research), like quercetin, suppress *H. pylori*.

Most ulcer sufferers simply accept the conventional antibiotic treatment for their ulcer because it works. The prescription drugs kill the bacteria and the ulcer heals, usually within two weeks, but with growing pressure on doctors to curtail the prescribing of these drugs and with so many patients increasingly concerned about the longer-term health risks of taking antibiotics, a cheap and natural alternative is certainly worth a try.

In his book *Vita-Nutrient*, Dr Robert Atkins, author, clinician and founder of the Atkins Center for Complementary Medicine in New York, describes a substance called gamma-oryzanol (isolated from rice bran oil) as, quite simply, The Ulcer Healer.

For the last two decades, Japanese scientists have been investigating this substance's healing properties for both gastric and cardiovascular complaints. (It has also been shown to help relieve menopausal symptoms and is commonly believed by bodybuilders to increase growth hormone secretion, but animal studies suggest this is not the case, and that it in fact inhibits the production of the growth hormone.)

In hundreds of hospital trials monitoring thousands of patients in the Far East, reseachers looked at recovery rates from gastrointestinal problems after taking conventional drug treatments or taking 300–600mg of gamma-oryzanol a day.

They found, without question, that the gamma-oryzanol users had better recovery rates than those taking the orthodox medications.

Another remedy finally getting the attention it deserves is mastic gum – which, as with so many alternatives, is anything but new. Highly prized in ancient Greece for its wide-ranging medicinal properties, it is the resin from the mastic tree (*Pistacia lenticus*) which grows only on the rocky slopes of Chios, a Greek island in the Aegean Sea, just off the coast of Turkey.

Used more commonly as a breath freshener, a flavouring in liquors and a stabiliser in paints, there was a time in the ancient world when the penalty for stealing mastic was amputation of the ears, nose or limbs. Today, thankfully, you can buy it in supplement form.

Laboratory tests have shown that mastic can kill at least seven strains of *H. pylori*. Clinical trials report that it can improve all symptoms in patients with ulcers. In one placebo-controlled trial, patients with medically-confirmed duodenal ulcers were given either 1 gram of mastic or a placebo every day for two weeks. An impressive 80% of those taking the mastic reported a definite improvement in their symptoms. In 70% of these happy patients, a re-examination of their ulcers by endoscope astounded doctors who found the previous ulcerations had been completely replaced by normal cells. Better still, nobody reported any side-effects.

Even in the minority of ulcers where *H. pylori* is not the main cause, mastic can help. In animal studies, its protective and healing effects have been demonstrated where the damage has been caused by aspirin ingestion or by other non-steroid anti-inflammatory drugs (NSAIDs), which are the second leading cause of ulcers.

While the mechanism for this miraculous cure remains unexplained, what researchers do know is that even relatively low doses of mastic gum – just 1mg a day for two weeks – can bring about a rapid cure of peptic ulcers.

I rarely used the word 'cure' since, in this field, it is all to easy to offer false hope. In fact, I cannot think of a single article in the thousands I have written on natural therapies for everyday conditions where I have suggested a remedy may even be a cure. On this occasion I am making an exception since the preliminary clinical trials really do hold great promise for those ulcer sufferers who are intolerant of or simply wishing to avoid antibiotics.

Vaginal Dryness

When a group of women suffering this problem were given a treatment plan which increased the amount of soya in their diet and supplemented their diet with linseed oil and red clover, doctors noticed that the vaginal tissues changed, for the better, in just 10 weeks. The results were reported in the *British Medical Journal*.

Linseed oil is an important source of essential fatty acids (EFAs) which lubricate the skin, joints and vaginal tissues. You can take this in liquid form but you can also get EFAs from nuts, seeds and oily fish. Vitamin E will also help. You need to take 300iu (international units) daily. For more direct action, you can insert the capsules into the vagina, where the body's heat will melt the outer casing and allow the nutrient to act where it is needed. If you do this, make sure you use a yeast-free preparation.

You need to be eating more of the plant phytoestrogens which have been found to help rebalance hormones in both sexes. GM-free organic soya is an excellent source. You can also supplement your diet with an American product called Pro-Estron (see Resources), which contains soy plus the hormone-balancing herb Agnus castus and the Chinese herb Dong Quai (which will rehydrate the vaginal tissues). You will also to need to take red clover, which will work fastest when taken in tincture form.

Varicose Veins

Varicose veins are caused by a weakness in the walls of the blood vessels. They are four times more common in women, will often develop during pregnancy and may also run in families. Haemorrhoids, which are usually the result of excessive straining during bowel movements due to constipation, are actually varicose veins in the anus and rectum, and so will respond to the same treatment. Both standing or sitting for long periods will exacerbate the problem, but herbs and supplements can be very successful in keeping the symptoms under control.

If you are absolutely sure your current problem is the result of varicosity, then Ginkgo biloba, now widely used to promote good circulation throughout the body, can bring the condition back under control and help prevent a recurrence. Vitamin E will also improve circulation to the outer extremities, including the legs. Rutin is one of the hundreds of bioflavanoids which give citrus fruits and orange and yellow vegetables their vivid colours. It works to improve the strength of the body's small blood vessels and capillaries, which, in turn, strengthens veins. Bilberry is even better. Its effects in the body are reported to be twice as strong and to last twice as long as rutin.

The herb Horse chestnut can be used both internally and externally to treat varicose veins. Early studies have shown that 300mg, three times a day will help. Constipation and lack of fibre in the diet are now believed to play an underlying role in the development of haemorrhoids (see Constipation, page 121). A salve made of white oak bark can also be used externally to soothe the pain.

Verrucae

Verrucae are simply warts on the soles of the feet, caused by a virus, which has invaded the skin and caused the cells to multiply rapidly and form raised lumps. The body cannot kill off the virus and so, instead, walls off these lumps, which are highly contagious. (Most children, for example, pick up verrucas from swimming pools and school changing rooms.) The constant pressure of walking on them causes them to harden and burrow deeper into the skin, which can, eventually, make walking painful.

Among the more bizarre remedies I have seen, but one that really can work for some people, is banana skin. You tape a small piece of very ripe (even blackened) banana skin to your foot, so that the inside surface is in contact with the verruca. The explanation lies in the fact there is an enzyme in the banana skin, which attacks the wart.

Verrucae are always a signal that your immune system is weakened, so take a good multivitamin. If you are treating children, find a multivitamin specifically formulated for their age group and make sure it does not have added artificial sweeteners, especially aspartame. Children (and animals) both respond fantastically well to homeopathic medicine. The remedy Causticum 6c can help get rid of this annoying infection.

Vitiligo

Vitiligo is a skin disorder characterised by the progressive and patchy enlargement of an area of de-pigmented (white) skin. It is caused by the destruction of melanocytes, the cells that produce the melanin pigment which darkens the skin, and is thought to affect up to 4% of the world's population.

Anecdotal evidence points to the herb St John's Wort, which, while more often used as a mild antidepressant, makes the skin more sensitive to light. If you do decide to try it, avoid red wine, cheese and yeast and consult a qualified herbalist to determine the correct dose for you. Another herb called khella has been found to help with vitiligo, but again it can have unpleasant side-effects, including nausea and insomnia, so take advice before self-prescribing.

Studies of people suffering vitiligo have shown low levels of folic acid, vitamin B_{12} and vitamin C. A treatment plan which included very high doses of folic acid plus 1g of vitamin C daily and intramuscular injections of vitamin B_{12}, carried out and supervised by a qualified health practitioner, produced a marked re-pigmentation in a small number of sufferers who stuck with this programme for several months.

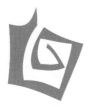

part three

Hands-on:

An A–Z of Selected

Complementary Therapies,

from Acupuncture to

Zero Balancing

Introduction

There are now over 100 complementary therapies. Some have their origins in the ancient healing traditions of Chinese or Ayurvedic medicine; others are relative newcomers, having been devised in the late 20th century. A number of them – such as floatation, the Bach Flower Remedies and zero balancing – have been discovered and brought to us by medically-trained doctors, but many have not.

The biggest problem in complementary medicine is that there are no real regulations. There is nothing to stop me, for example, doing a weekend course in Reiki and then opening a clinic and dealing with real patients. The second biggest problem is that too many people expect the same quick fix from their complementary health practitioner that they were disappointed not to get from their family physician.

As with all fields, there are excellent, good, average, poor and downright dangerous practitioners out there, so the risks are very real. This is not your car or your washing machine you are tinkering with, it is your health and the only body you have. There is nothing wrong with being a guinea pig, if you know that is what you are. Of course practitioners have to train, but if you do not want them training on you, you should be asking anyone who plans to treat you what qualifications they have, where they trained, how much clinical experience they have and how much experience of your particular complaint. Also check that they are a member of any of the established and recognised organisations that can give accreditation for their training.

Another mistake people make, especially when they book into a health spa, is to arrange for a series of complementary treatments, back to back. Just the thought of this gives me the shivers. If, for example, you have a holistic body massage, you should be taking your body off to bed to rest for a couple of hours, not rushing off down the corridor for a Shiatsu or Reiki treatment.

On the subject of Reiki, I have upset large numbers of practitioners in the past when I asked how it was possible to become a 'Master' of anything after a couple of weekend attunement courses. My postbag doubled with letters of complaint from Reiki practitioners, telling me how marvellous this therapy is and how it was clear I did not know the first thing about it.

It is true that I have not, to date, allowed any Reiki practitioner anywhere near me. This is not because I do not believe it works. Indeed, the opposite holds true. It is because I suspect it is a very powerful tool and that, in the wrong hands, you could really end up feeling worse.

I have acupunture once a fortnight and I try to have a zero balancing session once a month. I practise yoga and have two wonderful teachers, Fildema Spilsbury and Sue Pennington, who teach different styles. I meditate and I float whenever I can escape for a few hours. I have a kind of physical and mental MOT at the change of each season with an holistic skin therapist who practises Mora Therapy, and I tailor my vitamins and herbal supplements to my needs, according to her diagnosis. The reason I tell you this is because this is enough for me – you need to find out what's enough for *you*.

The success of any holistic healthcare programme lies, ultimately, with you. These therapies are not an antidote to junk diets, smoking, a sedentary lifestyle or even depression. They work to support you holistically, but the real work must come from you. That is why I like some of the more powerful and less obvious techniques, especially the Metamorphic Technique where a good practitioner will tell you, 'You do all the work, I just hold the energies.'

Even techniques that appear seemingly harmless, especially aromatherapy and reflexology, are very powerful. Make sure you only put your foot in someone's hands once you are sure they know what they are doing.

You expect your doctor to have passed exams, read the relevant scientific papers and to have kept abreast of developments in his or her field. Expect no less from your holistic practitioner.

In this section I have highlighted a range of the hands-on and healing therapies I often get asked to explain. There are, of course, many more and, as you will see, many variations on a theme. Kinesiology, for example, which is a very powerful diagnostic tool when practised by an expert, has 16 different schools. The one I have chosen to write about is one that seriously impressed me when I saw it in action on other people and experienced it myself. It rid me of a nagging predominantly muscular lower backpain, caused by sitting for too long at a computer terminal, and worked where other remedies, including acupuncture, had offered only temporary relief.

If I have not included your favourite therapy or the technique that healed you, please feel free to let me know (see Contact Details in Resources). If you are practising a little-known, relatively new therapy that I should know about, get in touch.

If you just want to get a real and unbiased feel for some of the more powerful healing techniques currently on offer, and to gain a better understanding of their physical, mental and (where relevant) spiritual benefits before you choose the right one for you, read on.

For details of how to find a practitioner in your area or how to train in any of these disciplines, see Resources. For further, more detailed reading on any of these treatments, see Bibliography.

Acupuncture

Meditate: 'To know is not to prove, nor to explain, but to accede to vision.'

Think about acupuncture and you'll picture someone lying passively on a couch with rows of tiny needles sticking out of their skin. The practitioner, presumably, has gone for a cup of antioxidant green tea. In fact, the first time I had acupuncture treatment, the needles were inserted in just two points – alongside the thumb and on the wrist – and then quickly removed. In China, practitioners do tend to leave the needles in. In the West, many will often use them to stimulate the flow of energy – which takes less than a fraction of a second – and then remove them.

Since acupuncture first arrived in the West in the late 1930s, it has become one of those therapies we have all heard of. This means we *think* we know what it is, until we actually try it for ourselves or study it. We've all heard stories of people undergoing major operations using acupuncture instead of anaesthetic, so we know it works. For most of us, we just don't know why or how.

Science has recently come on board following a well-publicised trial where researchers used a mock needle to investigate whether acupuncture really did make a difference or whether people just felt better thanks to the placebo effect.

The fake needles simulated the same experience of a treatment but, unlike the real thing, did not actually penetrate the skin. Volunteer patients were divided into two groups, but were not told who was getting a genuine acupuncture treatment and who was not.

The results, published in *New Scientist* magazine, showed a significant difference in the responses of the two groups of 52 volunteers, all of whom had presented with painful shoulder injuries. Each participant had been given eight 20-minute sessions over a period of four weeks. At the end of the trial, the number of real acupuncture recipients reporting a positive improvement in their symptoms was 40% higher than those who had been given the placebo or fake treatment. Similar controlled trials for different conditions are now planned; in the UK, half of all doctors now want acupuncture to be made available on the NHS.

The word acupuncture means 'to puncture with a needle' and, in simple terms, the needles are used to stimulate and rebalance the body's own healing energy or *chi* and to remove the blockages that are responsible for sickness and low energy. This is done by gently inserting fine, stainless steel and sterile needles at particular points on the body, which are themselves linked by energy channels or *meridians*.

There are 12 of these meridians. Each is connected to a specific organ in the body and each one has over 350 acupuncture points. As well as using needles, the practitioner may also use moxibustion. Here, a Chinese herb called 'Moxa' (*Artemesia vulgaris latiflora*), which is similar to mugwort, is shaped into a small cone that is placed on an acupuncture point and then lit to warm the body and stimulate *chi*. It feels wonderful and is said to stimulate blood flow, as well as *chi*.

At your first acupuncture session, the practitioner will take a detailed medical history and then ask to look at your tongue. This can be a bit embarrassing, but is a crucial part of the diagnosis. A pink, fleshy tongue is a sign of glowing good health. One that has a yellow or white coating carries the telltale signs of a system that is functioning below par. Different parts of the tongue also represent different systems in the body. The middle, for example, represents the stomach and the spleen. The back tells the practitioner about the state of your kidney, bladder and gut.

Your acupuncturist will then take your pulses – six at each wrist – to assess your physical, emotional and spiritual health. Again, these pulses relate to different organs in the body. A treatment can take between 30 minutes and an hour. The number of acupuncture points used will depend on the diagnosis, the patient's age, sensitivity, wellness and build.

During my first-ever acupuncture session, I could immediately feel the energy or *chi* moving in my body, but people's reactions to the stimulus of the needles will vary. People report different sensations during treatment. I usually feel a tiny prick when the needles first puncture the skin, followed by a dragging sensation as the energy flows to, from and around that point. Some people report feeling a surge of invigorating energy straight away. Some feel fatigued, and others describe the sensation as a deep dragging feeling towards the points where the needles have been placed. The chances are, the more holistic and toxin-free your lifestyle, the more sensitive your energy is and the more quickly your pulses will respond to the treatment.

You may not feel anything during a treatment; this is normal too. If you are worried or scared of the needles, what you need to know is that it does not usually hurt. You can even avoid looking at the needles by keeping your eyes closed, which will help you to stay relaxed.

You can use acupuncture to help you stop smoking, lose weight, treat migraines, lower blood pressure, relieve constipation and alleviate skin disorders. Obviously, the number of treatments you need will depend on your short- and longer-term goals. I have it, for example, to *stay* well; to help keep my energies balanced, to boost my immune system, remain centred in myself and strengthen my energy.

The extraordinary thing about acupuncture is that nobody can predict the changes it will trigger. This is because your body will do what it needs to do. For example, when I first went for a treatment session, I told the practitioner I had a history of digestive and skin problems which I had learned to control for the most part with diet. She, therefore, treated my large intestine and I spent a week running to the toilet. It was as if my body was having a clear-out – a kind of colonic irrigation without the embarrassment of that treatment. When my digestive system had settled down again, I then developed a sore throat. The throat is linked to the lungs, and my acupuncturist had, unbeknownst to me, also treated my lungs.

If you are a woman, one of the first and most profound changes acupuncture brings about can be the rebalancing of your hormones so that your menstrual cycle becomes regular again.

I now have acupuncture every fortnight and agree with my acupuncturist, Angela Hicks, who says: 'I don't know how people manage without acupuncture in their lives.'

The Alexander Technique

Good for: musculoskeletal problems, especially lower back pain; better posture and breathing troubles. It is popular among those involved in the performing arts, horseriders and musicians.

The whispered 'ahs' and deep 'monkey squats' that anyone who practises this technique will be familiar with were my first introduction to complementary health. In the mid-1980s I had the good fortune to meet and then share a flat with an Alexander Technique teacher called Rachel Stevens, who taught me how to find and then sit on my sitting bones. Back then, few people had even heard of this technique. Today, there are hundreds of teachers and it is widely available.

Less of a therapy and more of a re-education of how you move and use your body, the Technique not only improves posture but is excellent for a wide range of musculoskeletal problems, especially lower back problems.

It was devised by Frederick Mathias Alexander, an Australian actor who developed voice problems on stage. What he discovered, through a long process of detailed self-observation using mirrors, was that when asked to perform, he would tense his neck muscles. This then pulled his head back and down which, in turn, compressed his vocal cords. The movement was easy to miss, but once he had it pinpointed, he could see how it would have an impact on his voice. He learned how to correct this habit so that he did not lose his voice again. He then went on to develop this technique, which recognises the importance of maintaining a balanced relationship between the head, neck and spine, no matter what activity you are engaged in.

One very simple Alexander Technique exercise to learn and practise yourself is one which allows the spine to rest in a natural position. First, you need a small pile of books to rest your head on. These should be the equivalent, when stacked, of about 5cm or three-fingers' deep. To relax the spine completely, you lie on the floor with your knees bent upwards and your head resting on your books for 15 minutes.

An Alexander Technique lesson will last about 45 minutes. One of the wonderful benefits is that you can emerge about 1cm taller, and lots of people who practise this technique report that it makes them feel both taller and more elegant.

In a survey carried out to investigate this stretching phenomena, 10 healthy adults were given an Alexander Technique lesson, once a week, for 20 weeks. Another 10 equally healthy volunteers, matched for height, weight and sex, agreed to be the control group. After 20 weeks, those people who had received treatment were shown to have more respiratory muscular strength and greater levels of endurance than those who had not undergone the Technique.

The researchers concluded that these benefits were a result of the fact that the Alexander Technique stretches the torso.

At your first lesson, the postural habits you have acquired since childhood will be assessed. You will be asked to walk around the room and perform simple, everyday activities such as sitting and standing. You may also be treated while lying down on a couch, when the therapist will realign your body, stretch out your limbs and help you re-educate yourself on how to move and use your body more efficiently. Sheer bliss!

Aromatherapy

Good for: relaxation, combatting stress, promoting well-being and peace, insomnia, anxiety, depression, arthritis, supporting cancer treatments and improving the quality of hospice care.

Still the most popular and fastest-growing of all the hands-on complementary therapies, aromatherapy has introduced hundreds of thousands of people to the idea of taking better care of their health. In the nineties, sales of aromatherapy oils rocketed by 70%, and most people who have tried some form of complementary therapy have had aromatherapy.

Based on the healing properties of the essential plant oils that give different plants their unique smells, there are three types of aromatherapy. **Holistic aromatherapy** uses these essential oils together with massage to treat a wide range of physical and emotional disorders. **Clinical aromatherapy** integrates the technique with orthodox medical treatments, but is still not practised widely in the UK. **Aesthetic aromatherapy** is the one that is on offer in beauty salons. It is wonderfully relaxing and may even help with a number of skin disorders, but it is only one small aspect of this whole discipline.

There are few clinical trials proving the efficacy of aromatherapy, but those who have had this treatment are in no doubt that it works. The oils stimulate the sense of smell, which then affects that part of the brain known as the limbic system. This is connected to mood control, strong emotions and instinctual behaviour. Think about how smells not only remind you of certain places and events but of specific times in your life. I have a soothing sage face gel called

Panacea which I sometimes use with a lavender toner. I once took both products to a yoga retreat on a wonderful Greek island at the end of summer. Even today, I cannot use either of these without being transported straight back to that time.

The aromatherapy massage can itself release powerful emotions and tensions, so do not be surprised to find yourself wiped out but very relaxed after a treatment. You may have a mild adverse reaction, say a headache, but this will pass in a day or two.

Aromatherapy is now a popular treatment in hospitals, hospices and homes for the elderly. It can bring about feelings of great peace and pleasure, and is an excellent antidote to many of those conditions linked with older age, including depression, insomnia, anxiety and arthritis.

When 100 cardiac patients who had undergone surgery were randomly divided into four groups, those given proper aromatherapy treatments were found to be significantly calmer, less anxious and more relaxed than either those who were treated with dummy oils, those who were counselled by nurses and those who had no support at all.

If you have hypersensitive skin, you will need to be careful about which oils you use. You also need to learn how to dilute oils using a carrier base, since neat oils should never come into contact with the skin. If a therapist comes at you brandishing a bottle of essential oils and promising to get rid of your toxins, run a mile. This is not the point of aromatherapy.

If you have high blood pressure, epilepsy, skin disorders or if you are taking certain homoepathic medicines, you will need to avoid some oils. Never apply oil to areas of the skin which have been damaged or have open wounds. Some oils can be phototoxic, so check that it is safe to be out in the sun after a treatment. Others should not be used during pregnancy. Again, check the one you are planning to use is safe.

Astanga Yoga

Forget a gentle stretch class in a half-empty, unheated church hall with a lazy teacher. With astanga – pronounced ashtanga – yoga, you won't need the heating on anyway. This is the discipline that gave Madonna her fabulous post-pregnancy physique and, she says, a more compassionate outlook on life. It also explains the radiant good health and incredible equipoise of fellow superstar, Sting. So devoted are these two to the practice, they have, along with others, shared European summer holidays in Italy, where the presence of the resident astanga yoga teacher was more important than the pool.

Although not a therapy in the sense of a healer putting his or her hands on you, there is no doubt you will progress more quickly if you find a good teacher who will adjust your position to help you achieve and then hold the postures (or *asanas*) as you practise. Sharath Rangaswamy, the grandson of Sri Pattabhi Jois – whose devotees honour him with the title Guruji – is the natural heir to the astanga tradition in Mysore, India, where he teaches and where many of the world's best astanga teachers go to study themselves. He gets up at 2a.m. so he can do his own two-hour practice before teaching a pre-dawn daily class at 4.30a.m. and is famed for nudging people into the right position with his *bare feet*.

A decade ago, astanga yoga was almost unheard of outside India. Today it is the fastest-growing yoga discipline. Until recently it got a bad press, with people shying away from its macho but mistaken image. The name 'Power Yoga' did not help. It is true that with this type of yoga you do sweat and you do jump between positions, but the sweating is simply the result of the way the postures are dynamically linked (which means the body keeps moving) and the jumping is never compulsory and more like a bunnyhop. It can, of course, be macho, but only if you get the wrong teacher. If the idea of power in the context of a deeper connection, a stronger more fluid physique and a healthier psyche appeals, then this is the yoga for you. It will also, if you practise regularly, give you a flat stomach.

Astanga yoga differs from all other schools in that you deliberately heat the body first. The theory is that warmed muscles can stretch further and with more ease. You also learn a breathing or pranic technique called *ujjayi* breathing. In other forms of yoga this is taught, but used only in specific breathing exercises (Pranayama) or when the body needs help in releasing into a posture. It is a calming, cleansing breath which is said to confer more benefits than the postures themselves. It is a loud, audible breathing which is achieved by partially closing the back of the throat and sucking air in and out. The mouth stays closed and when you get the hang of it, it sounds, say teachers, like the ocean rolling on the shore. It provides an excellent focus for beginners confused by the postures or the sequences, and is fantastically soothing.

A class begins with two versions of the Sun Salutations. These are a series of postures linked dynamically and designed to warm the body up. You then work your way through the 55 postures in what is called the Primary or Healing First Series. For beginners, following a set sequence and not having to create your own practise programme frees you to concentrate on the breathing and the deeper aspects of your yoga, especially when you practise on your own.

Getting hot and sweaty during astanga practice is a good sign. When you start, you may also notice a peculiar smell, which you soon realise is coming from you. This is a good sign too. It shows the body is releasing deep-held toxins; this is a short-lived phase which quickly passes. The idea is to take your practice at your own pace. Once you have mastered the ujjayi breathing, you will soon find your yoga becomes like a moving meditation. Pay no attention to others in your class. The emphasis of astanga is self-practice, so do what feels right for you at the time. You will have more energy but feel more stiff if you practise in the mornings. In the evenings, you will be more flexible but more tired too, so adjust your practice accordingly. You can use a video or a CD (see Resources) to keep you motivated – or, better still, start your own self-practice group.

How much yoga you do is up to you. It is better to do a little each day than just one big session a week, but you must decide for yourself. You can go to class once a week or practise at home every day on your own. It is worth remembering that 10 minutes of practice is always worth a tonne of theory, but you may not want to make a daily commitment – in which case, aim to practise three times a week. You can practise for as long or as little time as you like, but always make sure you do the finishing poses, which counter earlier postures and keep the body balanced.

Remember, all yoga was originally designed to straighten the spine for meditation, so after your practice is an excellent time to meditate. Do not be tempted to skip the deep relaxation at the end. This is when the real regenerative work takes place, so try to relax completely for at least 10 minutes.

So, what changes can you expect? Lightness. Strength. Fluidity. Better concentration. A calmer and more compassionate outlook. Less fat. A flat stomach. Greater flexibility. The list goes on – and better still, once you have learned the basic moves from a good teacher, astanga yoga is completely free.

The Sun Salutations and the Primary Series are enough to keep you practising for a lifetime, but if you feel you wish to go further and deeper into the practice, there are the Second and Third (advanced) Series to look forward to. Most city-based teachers run drop-in daily classes, so you can come and go as you please.

With dedication, you will change your whole body shape, bring a deeper sense of peace and connectedness into your life and boost your health and vitality. Most regular practitioners, remember, look at least 10 years younger than their biological age!

Ayurveda

Meditate: 'Better surely, to light a candle than to curse the darkness.'

Very fashionable but utterly confusing to many of us in the West, Ayurveda is the name given to the ancient Indian science of life. It is said that these healing skills were brought to consciousness by Pantajali, the spiritual guru and sage who some say also brought the world yoga and the sacred Sanskrit language. Others say he never even existed.

True Ayurvedic healing will revolutionise not only what you eat but when. You learn how to change your habits depending on the season, your dominant body type (or *dosha*) and how, if you stay faithful to its original principles, you would use enemas and even deliberate vomiting to spring-clean your system and cleanse the body of accumulated toxins.

These last techniques are, of course, too powerful for most of us in the West. Thankfully there are practitioners outside India who live and work by the Ayurvedic principles but who have adapted them to make them more relevant to Western life. Traditionalists may not like what they see as a corruption of the traditional Ayurvedic practices, but these adaptations have already benefited many people in Europe and America, and have become so popular, it is clear they are here to stay.

The Ayurvedic practitioner will combine disciplines including nutrition, herbal medicine, aromatherapy and massage to rebalance the body and prevent disease. First, though, he or she will make an assessment of your *dosha* or energy-type.

There are just three types; Vata (air), Pitta (fire) and Kapha (earth); once you know the key characteristics it is easy to determine not only your own dominant dosha but that of your family and friends too. The experienced eye can even tell just by looking at somebody. Newcomers will need more information – including, say, how they feel and how they react to certain foods.

Vata means 'to move' or 'to enthuse'. Vata people have agile minds, a lively imagination and a lot of get-up-and-go, but they can be guilty of over-indulgence and can burn out. Signs of disturbed Vata include arthritis, constipation, rheumatic pains, abnormal blood pressure and mental problems.

Pitta means 'to heat' or 'to burn'. Pitta people are clever and articulate. They are also irritable and proud. If you know someone whose hair went grey early, the chances are they are Pitta. They also have hot and sweatier bodies. Some skin disorders, anger, a yellow colouring to the skin, urine, faeces and eyes, and any burning sensations on the body are all signs that the Pitta energy is out of balance.

Kapha means 'to embrace' or keep together. Kapha people have patient, stable personalities and are slow to get angry. They are not easy to provoke but, once enraged, take a long time to calm down again. They are slow talkers and may be inclined towards lethargy and laziness. Flabby muscles, tiredness, impotence, feeling weak and feeling run down are all signals that the Kapha dosha needs rebalancing.

Don't worry if you don't like the dosha that best describes you. We all have all three energies, but one tends to dominate. Your Ayurvedic practitioner will also take account of the season and the climate you live in before prescribing treatment. One of the best ideas we can thank Ayurvedic medicine for is that of a start-of-the-season kind of holistic MOT where the body is detoxed and prepared for the new season ahead.

Massage treatments are an important part of Ayurvedic medicine. For sheer bliss and relaxation it would be hard to beat such soothing treatments, where, for example, warm oil is gently poured in a slow dynamic movement across the brow and in the region of the mystical Third Eye or the four-handed massage, where two therapists work in tandem with litres of detoxifying sesame oil which they massage into every part of the body. If you can overcome your shyness (since you need to be naked for this), you will think you have died and gone to Ayurvedic heaven!

The Bowen Technique

The Bowen Technique is a method of manipulating muscles which has achieved good results with musculoskeletal conditions, especially frozen shoulder and tennis elbow. It is another of those 'hard-to-explain-just-exactly-what-is-going-on' therapies, but what is clear is that it really works.

In fact, for the kind of problems that would usually be treated with cortisone injections, physiotherapy or surgery, it claims an impressive 70% recovery rate.

The idea is that the therapist tunes in to the specific health problem and triggers the body's own healing mechanism. During a treatment session, the practitioner will run his or her fingers and thumbs across the muscles, tendons and ligaments of the affected area with no more pressure than could be applied to an eyeball. These movements are like a 'roll' which disturbs the muscle enough to create an energy surge. The treated area is then left alone to assimilate and react to this disturbance.

Nobody really knows how or why this technique works. One idea is that it triggers a little-known communication system between the body's cells and the brain, which then organises the repair of damaged tissue or, in the case of tennis elbow, the damaged tendons.

The people I have witnessed being treated this way report a feeling of deep, peaceful relaxation after a session, and it is extraordinary to see the body react – you see a red welt-like mark appear where the pressure has been applied, although the technique is completely painless.

The first-ever study into the effectiveness of this technique on a specific condition – in this case, frozen shoulder – was carried out in the UK by the European College of Bowen Studies. Ironically, the pain associated with this problem itself exacerbates the condition, since the more reluctant the sufferer is to use the shoulder, the more it stiffens.

Over 3,000 volunteers called up asking to join the research programme. Patients were randomly assigned to a placebo-control group or to the treated group who were given three Bowen Technique treatments over a six-week period. The trial was blind, which means patients did not know which treatment they were getting. All patients were asked not to make lifestyle changes which might have affected the outcome over the study period.

None of the patients had been treated by a Bowen therapist before the study, and both groups were given exactly the same aftercare. What the researchers found was that those patients who had Bowen treatments improved significantly more than those who were in the placebo group. Almost 80% of those having Bowen sessions said their shoulder had improved. Only 20% of those in the placebo group could claim the same. About half of those in the placebo control said their shoulder had become worse over the six-week trial period. Fewer than 10% of the treated group complained that their condition had worsened.

As with so many of these hands-on therapies, the outcome of any treatment will depend on your own commitment to the programme and the skills of your therapist.

Chakra Healing

Good for: your overall well-being; recognising potential problem areas where energy may be blocked.

I would steer clear of most healers or therapists offering to take a wad of your cash to 'balance your chakras' over a weekend workshop. Quite simply, this is not a task anyone else can do for you, and while the chakras are important to your physical, emotional and spiritual health, most of us will spend a lifetime just learning how to tune in to our own energy centres which the yogis call Chakras.

Chakra healing has become deeply fashionable, coinciding with a massive surge of interest in all types of yoga in the West. The growing awareness of these important energy points is good, but the best way to find out about your chakras is to sit quietly in a meditative position and experience them for yourself.

Most people deal with seven energy centres, although some shamanic practitioners recognise nine, including one below the feet (in the ground) and one above the head in the auric field. Here, we will concentrate on the seven better-known chakras.

Two of these, the crown and the brow chakras, are in the head. The remaining five follow the route of the spinal column from the base to the throat. When tuning in to your chakric energy, always start at the bottom and work your way up.

I find the easiest way to do this is to imagine energy flowing up from the ground through your feet and legs to the first or base chakra, which can also be called the root chakra. You may be imagining a straight line or have trouble feeling anything at all but this energy travels in a spiral motion so this image, which is closer to what is actually going on, may help.

The **root chakra** is at the base of the spine where the coccyx lies. It is said to be red in colour and concerned with matters relating to the material world. It has to do with grounding, stillness, courage and health, as well as your individuality.

Only experience can really tell you whether a chakra energy centre is blocked, open or closed, but the physical body can provide some clues. If, for example, you get a headache when you feel overloaded, it is your sixth or brow chakra, which is also known as the mystical Third Eye, that is being affected. If you feel a frog or tightness at the back of your throat, there is a blockage with the throat chakra there.

You will find the **second chakra** in the lower abdominal area, just below the navel. This is orange and is linked with procreation, your sexuality, how you digest and eliminate your food and your vitality. It is also linked to your health and feelings of desire and pleasure. The wise men say that this is the chakra most Western people are operating from. It is the dominant chakra for most Western men when they have sex; women tend to operate from the next chakra, which is called the solar plexus, or even the one above that – the heart chakra.

The **solar plexus chakra** is yellow and linked with the element of fire. It vitalises the metabolic and digestive processes and the emotions. It is linked with laughter and a love of life, and is all about learning to master ourselves and control our will.

The green **heart chakra** needs no introduction since it is clearly going to be about unconditional love, forgiveness, acceptance, peace and harmony. It energises the physical body and the blood with the power of the life-force and is concerned with the lungs and the circulation.

The blue **throat chakra** is the chakra of communication. If you have ever started to say something that you know you should probably keep to yourself and felt your throat constrict as you've done so, then you have already felt your throat chakra at work. It is linked with the power of expression, with learning how to use knowledge wisely and with the qualities of gentleness and kindness.

Most people have heard of something called the mystical Third Eye; this is the point at the centre of the brow, midway between the eyes, the site of the **brow chakra**. The colour is indigo or dark blue. This centre, when balanced and open, is about intuition, insight, imagination, peace of mind and, often, clairvoyance. Wisdom, devotion and a realisation of the presence of the soul are all linked with this energy centre, which is often the focus of meditation for practitioners. The last energy centre we will deal with here is the **crown chakra**, right at the top of the head. This vitalises the upper brain and is concerned with spiritual lessons and realisations, including the unification of the higher self with the personality, unity and divinity.

To check in with your own chakras and energy flow, sit quietly in a chair with your back straight, feet placed flat on the floor. Close your eyes and try to feel the energy moving up towards the root chakra. Rest your attention there, imagine the vivid red colour and see what images or notions come into your mind. These may hold clues about the state of this chakra and your journey through this world. Practise 'tracking' your energy up through all seven chakra centres and slowly back again, down through the centre of the body until you discharge the energy back to the ground. This simple exercise will tell you more about your physical, mental and spiritual well-being than any weekend workshop healer. It gets easier each time you do it, and is an excellent way to meditate and check in with yourself.

Cranial Osteopathy

Good for: Back, neck and shoulder pain during pregnancy, migraines, whiplash injuries, stomach ulcers, circulatory problems, breathing troubles and sluggishness. After a difficult labour, cranial osteopathy can greatly help both the mother and baby, especially if they are in shock.

Osteopathy focuses on the structural and mechanical workings of the musculoskeletal system. Cranial osteopathy, as the name suggests, brings that focus even tighter and concentrates solely on the skull.

The underlying principle of osteopathy is that structure governs function and vice versa. If you accept these two systems are completely dependent on each other then you will also accept that if you throw one out, you will affect the workings of the other.

The osteopath relies on gentle manipulation to ensure that the circulation of both the blood and the waste-removing lymph is balanced. This then helps the body fight disease and correct problems using its own healing powers. The treatment also helps remove toxins, since the lymphatic system, which has no pump, relies on exactly this type of movement to keep functioning.

Cranial osteopathy, then, ensures that the circulation of the cerebral spinal fluid in the skull is unimpeded so that the body can truly relax and rebalance itself. The therapist manipulates the bones of the skull and face to this effect. The technique is so gentle that it is hugely popular with stressed-out mothers, who say it works wonders with babies who do not sleep and children who are bunged up with ear, nose and throat problems.

Many women also report benefits when they have this technique following a difficult labour.

Cranial osteopathy was developed by Dr William G. Sutherland (1873–1954) who believed you could view life as a series of pulsating contractions and expansions which he called 'the breath of life'. According to him, a healthy cranosacral system pulsates at the rate of between 6 and 15 times a minute. Until his work, doctors and others believed the bones in the face and skull were fixed. Dr Sutherland showed how, in fact, they were capable of minute movements and could be manipulated into a proper healthy balance to correct that pulse.

Crystal Therapy

I have to admit I was sceptical – until Dutch-born Lettie Vantol, who runs the Vantol College of Crystal Therapy in the UK, got her hands on me. She warned, as she carefully placed crystals around my body, that most people feel no effects until the following day. She was right. I woke the next morning feeling sick and spent the better part of the day wondering if I was going to throw up.

The problem, at that time, was clearly one of liver congestion, and I was shocked by how powerful and deep-acting I found this hands-on therapy, which many still consider a bizarre, fringe technique.

The treatment itself feels quite extraordinary and, if you know what happens when you meditate, produces very similar results. You lie on the treatment couch and as your body starts to feel heavier, so do the crystals that have been placed on or alongside various body parts to stimulate the internal flow of energy and to unblock those parts where this energy has become stuck.

By the end of my first session, which lasted about an hour and during which I thought, at one point, I was in danger of spiralling quite happily off into the astral plane (I later discovered Vantol was using calcite, which some claim facilitates this), I felt unable to move my arms or legs.

Crystal therapy has been one of the latest of the 'fringe' treatments to move into more mainstream healing. What I learned from my experience with one of the UK's leading practitioners is that, in the right hands, it is a powerful tool. That said, and because of this potency, I would not want any old therapist or someone fresh from a weekend course brandishing even a seemingly harmless rose quartz crystal in my direction.

Crystals in this type of healing are used to help the body initiate its own deep healing processes, and while the technique may be perceived as being relatively new, the use of crystals, said to be a source of life and energy, is one of the oldest known practices in healing rituals. The shaman 'medicine men', for instance, used crystals in soul healing, as did the Aborigines, who went so far as to sew crystals under the skin.

Different crystals are assigned different healing properties. Turquoise, for example, was used by the ancient Egyptians to treat cataracts and eye problems. Calming and peaceful, its high copper content makes it a good conductor of energy; it is also used to revitalise the blood, tone the body and encourage tissue regeneration for wound-healing.

Red garnet is used for strengthening the heart, thyroid, liver and kidneys, and can help ease nausea, especially during a detoxification programme. Calcite is used to reduce stress and to ground excess energy, while rose quartz, one of the most popular crystals (and known as the Love Stone), has a positive effect on the kidneys and the ciruclation, as well as enhancing fertility.

Lettie Vantol, who comes from a long line of healers, agreed when I told her I would not want to be treated with crystals by someone who was not sure of what they were doing: 'Crystals are the strongest tool for healing that I have come across. You want to avoid being treated by someone who is just dabbling in them,' she warned.

Crystals are powerful because they work with your own energy, so if you buy one, make sure you cleanse it by leaving it for three days in pure water. Let it dry naturally and don't let anyone else touch it.

Not for beginners or dabblers. In the wrong hands this could cause more harm than good, so find someone who knows exactly what they are doing.

The Feldenkrais Method

Good for: back pain, neck tension, musculoskeletal complaints, poor digestion, insomnia, mental alertness and improved flexibility.

If you like the idea of moving through life with minimum effort and maximum efficiency, this is the system for you. Developed by the Russian-Israeli scientist Dr Moshe Feldenkrais, who had a background in physics and engineering, it is not about striving to achieve goals but about moving and breathing with less effort and less tension.

The underlying theory is that if you can correct poor habits in the way you move and use your body, you can improve both your self-image and your overall health. It may sound like a gentle technique, but be warned, it can be demanding. Having said that, it definitely gets results.

The Feldenkrais Method is taught in two steps. First, you have a one-to-one lesson with a trained practitioner who uses touch to show you how you can improve both your breathing and movements. This is called a Functional Integration lesson. In the second phase, known as Awareness Through Movement, you will be taught in your lessons how to correct improper movements and habits through a series of gentle exercises that revolve around sitting and walking. This phase is usually taught in a group class, and takes effect through a kind of postural patterning where the body is re-educated through the repetition of the corrections.

Feldenkrais himself began to study the mechanics of human movement when an old knee injury, suffered during a game of football in his youth, started to play up. He discovered that just as the brain tells the body what to do, the body can tell the brain about the easiest and most effective ways to move.

Although improved posture is an obvious benefit, the Feldenkrais Method is not about posture, but function. You will learn how each part of your body moves in relation to the other parts, and how to become conscious of your breathing while you move. The idea is to learn for yourself how less is more and how, if you make less effort, you can become more sensitive to and in tune with your body and its needs.

Flower Remedies

Good for: emotional and stress-related problems

My first-ever introduction to any kind of herbal medicine was with a small, brown bottle of Rescue Remedy. This is, of course, probably the most famous of the 38 Bach Flower Remedies, which were originated by Dr Edward Bach, a Harley Street doctor and homeopath, in England in the 1930s. Today, they are used all over the world.

Bach may have been the beginning, but there are now so many flower remedies, if you are interested in learning more about this type of healing you are going to be spoiled for choice. American healer Richard Katz added another 100 remedies to the original Bach ones, and since then remedies from all over the world, including the essences of Sea Plants, have been produced. There are remedies that have been invigorated by sunlight, and remedies made by moonlight. You may want to try the essences that come from the Australian Bush or the rainforest. There are Angel flower remedies and even Alaskan ones.

There are no clinical studies to prove whether flower remedies work, and scientific analysis of a remedy will tell you it contains alcohol and water only. But many practitioners, who usually prescribe flower remedies alongside a hands-on technique such as kinesiology, are convinced they work. One of my favourite books on using flower essences successfully is called *The Lazy Person's Guide to Emotional Healing* and is written by British doctor, Andrew Tresidder, whose lucky patients cannot get enough of his flower healing.

When you embark on healing with flower essences, keep in mind that they are the catalysts for change in your life. The theory is that these remedies capture the true essence of a flower – the most highly evolved part of a plant – in water, which then contains a healing vibration which can bring about transformation on an emotional, spiritual and mental level. The flowers are taken from wild plants, bushes and trees and are then prepared in a special way which usually includes being left out in a crystal bowl full of spring water in sunlight, a method said to potentiate the remedy. It is this liquid which is diluted down many times and preserved in brandy to be sold commercially.

One of the joys of flower remedies is that they are completely safe, making them a wonderful introduction to complementary healing. They work on a vibrational level and transform negative emotions into positive ones. You can mix different remedies to create the right essence for a particular mood. One of my favourites is Dr Tressider's Bitch Mix, which contains holly, Impatiens (Busy Lizzy), pine, vine and willow to help soothe a frayed and irritable pre-menstrual temper, and his Relationship Mix, which has gentian, heather, chicory, walnut, red chestnut and other essences to encourage honest communication and forgiveness in partnerships.

To make your own combinations, you fill a 30ml dropper bottle with 9 parts of fresh (but not boiled) water and 1 part brandy to preserve the mixture. Add just 3 drops each of your chosen remedies and replace the top. Keep in mind, the whole time you are making your essence, what it is you want it to help you achieve or heal. To take the remedy, drop 2–3 drops onto your tongue, 4–6 times a day for up to six weeks. If you are avoiding alcohol, drop the essences onto your wrists, instead of your tongue.

Hypnotherapy

Good for: acute and chronic pain, emotional problems including stress, eating disorders, substance addiction, panic attacks, migraines, jet lag, phobias, sexual dysfunction and fertility, sleep problems and sports injuries ... but only in the right hands

One of the oddest things about hypnotherapy is that all too often people walk away from the therapist's couch not knowing whether they have been hypnotised or not. I cannot think of any other treatment where you may not be sure if you have indeed had the treatment or made it all up in your mind.

One of the problems is that most people's introduction to hypnotherapy is through a TV or stage show designed to humiliate the maximum number of people for the audience's entertainment. As Robert Farago, one of the world's leading health-orientated hypnotherapists, is fond of saying: 'How can you heal during the day and then use the same tool to humiliate at night?'

There is nothing wishy-washy or even New Agey about this practitioner, who calls himself a Command Hypnotherapist. After a session with Farago, you will not have to ask yourself, 'was I hypnotised? did it work?' You will know.

One of his tests (and he is usually quite reluctant to do this, since it puts a strain on him and the client) is a physical one. Before hypnosis, he will ask you to resist his attempts to lower your outstretched arm. Farago is a big man, and you know you are on a hiding to nothing – until, that is, he asks you to do the same thing under hypnosis.

After being taken into a hypnotic state, my arm did not budge, no matter how hard Farago pushed. He used all his weight in vain. My arm, which had given way so easily before hypnosis, remained rigid and firmly in place. It also ached for several days afterwards!

Lots of people are still very suspicious about hypnosis, and quite rightly so. The entire field is unregulated and there are far too many inexperienced practitioners dying to get their hands on you. Do not take pot luck with the practitioner you choose. Trust is a crucial part of the healing process, especially when hypnosis is involved, so if you don't like the hypnotherapist find someone else – and if, after one session, you have to ask 'Was I Hypnotised?', ask for your money back.

Everyone knows you can use hypnosis to break addictions and to tackle eating disorders, but one of its most valuable roles is in unravelling the true causes of those conditions where the subconscious appears to gain control, especially panic attacks.

It also gets excellent results in treating infertility, especially among older career women who have postponed starting a family and who may, deep in their subconscious, have an ambivalence about turning their lives upside down with a new baby.

Indian Head Massage

You'll have to plough through a lot of words, in this book and others, to find a therapy I dislike as much as this one. That does not mean it does not work. It just means it is not right for me. I've been prodded, nudged, needled, covered with colourful crystals, thumped, rolled and had my flesh squeezed, all in the name of research, but I have not yet come across another hands-on treatment that disconcerted me as much as this one.

Of course, as with all these therapies, you are, literally, in the hands of the practitioner. I hated my first Indian head massage, and so booked another, with a different therapist, to make sure it was not a personality clash. I hated the second one too, but as I say, that does not mean it will not be right for you.

In India, the head massage is hugely popular. Practised mostly by women, it massages the scalp, face, neck, shoulders, upper arms and upper back. You may prefer to strip down to your underclothes (above the waist), but this is not crucial and this is a massage that can be carried out in the workplace.

Practitioners are trained to follow a set sequence of movements which uses their thumbs, the fingertips, and the pads, heels and, at times, the whole of their hands.

The first part of the massage is designed to invigorate and stimulate, the second phase concentrates on relaxation and healing, paying special attention to the mystical Third Eye chakra in the middle of the forehead.

Lots of devotees describe this massage as sheer bliss, especially when combined with essential oils which nourish the hair and scalp and promote well-being. As I say, I simply found it agitating.

I do, though, know students who swear by it before exams, and it is true that one of the benefits, when it does work for you, is that it clears the head and sharpens the mind. Said to improve concentration, it can also relieve tension headaches and eye strain, and so is popular among office workers.

Iridology

Good for: can be a useful tool in the diagnosis of a range of conditions but, as we have seen with other techniques, only in a good practitioner's hands

I was deeply sceptical the first time an iridologist looked me straight in the eye – until, that is, she diagnosed an underlying condition it had taken doctors six years to identify. I think, as with all of these complementary therapies, the effectiveness of this technique, which is actually a tool for diagnosis, depends on the skill and experience of the practitioner.

The theory is that it is in the eyes that the nervous system comes to the surface. The iridologist believes that the nerve filaments of the iris are linked to every organ in the body. There is no anatomical evidence for this, but skilled practitioners maintain they can see not only your current state of health but also past conditions and future tendencies.

Hippocrates, the father of modern medicine, wrote about the significance of the markings of the eyes, and an iridologst will make a diagnosis that is also based on the shape, purity and the brightness of the colouring of the iris. In very general terms, white marks are said to indicate inflammation and overstimulation of a particular organ and may be a sign of ongoing healing, while darker marks are a sign of reduced function and understimulation.

The iris was properly mapped out in the 1950s by the American naturopath and author, Dr Bernard Jensen. He divided it into six zones or rings. The innermost ring is said to correspond to the stomach, the second to the large and small intestine, the third to the circulation of the blood and lymph, the fourth to the organs and hormone-producing endocrine system, and the fifth to the musculoskeletal system. The outermost ring is said to correspond to the skin and the organs of elimination.

The idea is that once a health problem has been confirmed or identified, the practitioner can then prescribe the nutritional or herbal remedies needed to correct it.

Unfortunately for iridology, when mainstream researchers decided to investigate its usefulness as a diagnostic tool it failed spectacularly. In a controlled environment, three iridologists were given photographs of the irises of patients with severe and moderate renal disease. The practitioners were not told of the underlying condition, and none of them was able to diagnose it with any degree of accuracy.

This brings me back to my initial observation about this technique, which is that it is a fantastic tool in the right hands – and utterly useless, if not downright dangerous, in the wrong ones.

Warning: Anyone with epilepsy should avoid this treatment, since the bright light used to make an assessment may cause problems.

Kinesiology

If you've only ever come across what I have heard referred to as 'One-armed Bandit' practitioners, you may have a somewhat warped view of kinesiology. These 'bandits' are the half-trained (and often half-brained) would-be healers who come at you, threatening to diagnosis your health problems by testing the muscles in your left or right arm. It might work, but it is a sorry introduction to a potent technique that actually has some 16 variations to its name.

I was more lucky, in that my own introduction to this hands-on therapy came from a very experienced UK practitioner, John Logue. A trainer with the Academy of Systematic Kinesiology and a former structural engineer, it was immediately clear he understood the workings of the body – inside and out – better than many inexperienced young doctors. Better still, the treatment banished a nagging lower back pain that had come on suddenly, for no apparent reason, and which I had been putting up with for several months.

In simple terms, kinesiology is a way of communicating directly with the body through a sequence of muscle tests, to find out just exactly what is going on. It is one of the least intrusive and best diagnostic tools in complementary health. I've seen practitioners in training sessions identify, for example, adult onset diabetes and extreme depression without asking the client a single question – just by testing the muscles.

Kinesiology takes the guesswork out of making a diagnosis and, in my view, should be a compulsory training course for all alternative health practitioners, not least because it provides an excellent understanding of the anatomy and physiology of the human body, as well as an introduction to its energetic patterns.

I was surprised, then, to learn that kinesiology has its roots, not in any Eastern healing tradition, but in the insurance industry. Insurance claims, to be exact. It evolved from the motion tests devised by insurers for doctors and other specialists to test personal injury claimants following accidents. In other words, these were tests carried out to see if people were lying about the extent of their injuries.

Today, kinesiology combines muscle testing with the principles of Traditional Chinese Medicine. Instead of using acupuncture needles, practitioners use touch. They believe their tests can identify food allergies and sensitivities, vitamin and mineral deficiencies, lymphatic and circulatory problems and even emotional blocks. Muscle weaknesses caused by these problems and an accumulation of toxins can then be identified and corrected, leading to improved posture, pain relief and better energy flow.

The founding father of kinesiology back in the early 1960s was a US chiropractor called Dr George Goodheart. He set about investigating why it was he could identify a problem, correct it and relieve the muscle strain during the time he had the client on the couch but how he could never get these pain-relieving corrections to 'stick'.

During his research Dr Goodheart discovered, by accident, that rubbing certain muscles did seem to get the body to hold on to the muscular corrections he had made. It turned out that it was not the muscle he was rubbing which held the key to subsequent pain relief, but what are known as the lymph sites.

The human body has eight pints of oxygen- and nutrient-carrying blood circulating around. It has twice that amount of waste-disposal lymph, which clears the blood and removes lactic acid from the muscles (this lactic acid can otherwise cause aches and pains). While blood is pumped around the body by the heart, the lymph system must rely on the body's own movements to maintain its flow through a series of one-way valves or glands. Stagnant lymph, with its accumulating waste products and toxins, is now believed to be at the root of more health problems than almost any other underlying cause.

What kinesiologists have discovered is that you can use the body's own muscles to find out what is happening with the lymphatic drainage, what state of health the internal organs are in, how the blood supply to the brain is at the time of testing and how the key energies are doing. You can then make adjustments to rebalance any of these factors.

For a treatment session, you lie on a therapy couch and move your limbs as directed. (If you are female, you may feel more comfortable wearing trousers.) During a demonstration session, and having told the practitioner about my back problem, I was asked to push against pressure he was exerting on my leg. I was not able to resist the force he was applying and he moved my leg easily. I was then shown how to stimulate the relevant lymph point, just up from the navel, by pushing it with my own fingers. When I did apply pressure at that point, my leg could easily resist the pressure it had given way under before.

Kinesiologists have a golden rule of thumb – 'Where it is is where it is not.' So, when I said I had nagging lower back pain, the practitioner manipulated my head and neck to relieve it. Like I said, it worked and it did not hurt. I felt some discomfort at the lymph point, but nothing that would stop me getting back on the treatment couch of an experienced practitioner. When my head was moved and manipulated, I simply felt relief. You keep your clothes on throughout the treatment, and what I liked was the fact that it was simple, quick, gentle, effective and completely non-intrusive.

John Logue, who practises in the UK but who trains and lectures worldwide, has produced an introductory leaflet to Systematic Kinesiology called *Seeing is Believing*. He knows most of us will not accept that what looks like prodding a muscle here and poking a lymph spot there really can cure such a wide range of ailments, from asthma to depression, backpain to migraines and chronic fatigue to phobias.

'With kinesiology, the body tells you exactly what is wrong and what it needs to be fixed. You cannot not help your client to get better. This system looks at the entire person and so is holistic in the truest sense,' he explains.

He admits, though, that he too is alarmed by what he calls the one-armed bandits – those health practitioners who have only a little knowledge of kinesiology but who use it anyway, relying on their limited ability to test just the one group of muscles in your outstretched arm while looking for signs of food sensitivities, nutritional deficiencies and other problems.

Once you know what is causing your health problems, you need to know what to do to get better, so if you are looking for a kinesiologist, find one who has a background in nutrition too. They can then recommend the best nutrients (such as vitamin E for backpain, chromium for insulin-dependent diabetes) for you to take. Do not expect an overnight cure. It usually takes between three and six treatment sessions before you feel a lasting improvement in your health.

For details of practitioners and charges, see Resources.

KOSMED/SCENAR

Developed behind closed doors by Russian scientists and used during the Cold War to keep their astronauts in peak physical condition, the KOSMED device looks like a slim, black TV remote control.

Now approved for pain relief in the UK, where it is undergoing hospital trials, it is also known as SCENAR – which stands for Self Controlled Energo Neuro Adapative Regulation. For the sake of simplicity, we will stick with the name KOSMED, which was chosen to stand for Cosmic Medicine. This does not mean I favour one or the other of the brand names (there is a lot of political infighting around this device), I just find KOSMED a more user-friendly name.

In Russia, where KOSMED is now used full-time by some 600 Russian practitioners and part-time by another 3,000 healers, incuding many doctors, the device won its makers the prestigious Order of Lenin award. It is, in essence, a biofeedback device, said to trigger the body's natural and potent healing powers by setting up a 'dialogue' between the brain and whichever part of the body or system needs healing.

It is said to work by sending a low-energy, nerve-like and painless electronic impulse through the skin. This signal then changes according to how the skin reacts. It is these changes which the KOSMED healer has been trained to interpret. All you will feel is a gentle tingle through the skin, but what you will see – if there is any underlying health problem or disturbance – can be as dramatic as a complete change in the colour of the skin tone, say from white to red, or a change to its texture, so that where it was smooth, it then feels sticky.

The idea is that the KOSMED, having detected the problem, alerts the brain to the affected area, thus reminding the body's own repair mechanisms to finish the healing job it may have started but not yet finished. Witnessing this treatment reminded me of the Bowen Technique (see page 275), whose practitioners use their fingers to trigger a similar reorganisation of the body's energy to encourage a natural repair job. The main difference between the two techniques is that the hands-on Bowen healers admit they do not really know how their treatment works.

What the Russian researchers discovered was that they could trigger the body's own powers of self-healing by stimulating the C-fibres of the neural network. These make up 70% of this network, but are much slower to conduct messages than the so-called A-fibres, which are the named nerves that supply the muscles. Where A-fibres are covered in a myelinated sheath which promotes faster conductivity, C-fibres are unsheathed.

The C-fibres are responsible for general cell maintenance and are used by the body to deliver its own pharmaceutical messages, in the form of proteins called *neuropeptides*. This means that healing chemicals can be produced where they are needed. A good analogy is to think of a printer which has been loaded with paper but which has not yet been sent a message of what to print. The KOSMED delivers that message and effectively tells the C-fibres what needs to happen, energetically and pharmaceutically, to finish the healing process.

A KOSMED treatment may last between 20 minutes and an hour. You book a series of treatments; the number will depend, of course, on the type and severity of your complaint. For PMT, for example, you would have a treatment session every day for say, seven days before your period and then every day for seven days after the last day of menstruation.

Although its approval by the authorities in the UK is for pain relief only, stories of astonishing and unlikely cures have been filtering through, causing a wave of excitement in healing circles. They include the overnight disappearance of an ovarian cyst the size of a grapefruit in one woman, and the repair of blood vessels to the foot of a man who was, until he had the KOSMED treatment, facing amputation. It has even been shown to completely repair old scar tissue.

Perfect healing, of course, would not leave a permanent scar, which serves no function for the body but is simply a sign, say KOSMED practitioners, of an electromagnetic disturbance now held as a 'memory' in the body's tissues. A scar also shows how the natural healing process has become 'stuck'.

What the Russians have discovered is that the body creates a special electrical team of cells and messages to carry out a repair job and then, when it thinks a good enough job has been done, disbands this team. These are the cells that KOSMED talks to and triggers to finish the job properly.

The theory is that the widespread use of this exceptional device could save countries billions in medical costs. It is a device that encourages people to keep well, instead of trying to salvage their health once they have fallen sick.

For KOSMED to work, though, you need three key ingredients: the patient's own willingness to recover completely, the device itself, and the practitioner's skill in using KOSMED and interpreting the readings, displayed as ever-changing numbers in the display window of the device. When this triangle works, it facilitates the body's own internal pharmacy to refine its repair work.

McTimoney Chiropractice

Good for: anyone who is nervous about having their bones manipulated; pain relief, musculoskeletal problems and, most of all, back pain

So gentle that animals and children love it, the McTimoney technique is another variation on the chiropractice theme and is perfect for anyone who is nervous about having their spine manipulated. Even lighter is the McTimoney-Corley version, where practitioners use only their fingertips to adjust the vertebrae gently. The perfect antidote to any kind of stress, it is also popular with the elderly and the very sick.

The technique is named after John McTimoney, a chiropractor working in the 1950s who promoted the idea that chiropractice should be used to treat the whole person and not just the area of the body that is causing some kind of musculoskeletal problem.

He believed that all parts of the body – the skull, the spine, the pelvis and the limbs – could lose their natural alignment, but that you need only the gentlest of measures to correct them.

McTimoney practitioners learn a technique called the 'toggle-torque-recoil' which they perform on the bones of the spinal column. The adjustments that are made with this method are very precise and very fast, so there is the minimum amount of discomfort for the patient.

You will not hear the tell-tale cracking sound of other forms of chiropractice (this, by the way, is not the noise of bones cracking but is caused when the gas bubbles present in the synovial fluid, which lubricates the joints, burst under pressure). McTimoney is so light, the patient may feel nothing at all. That does not mean there is nothing going on. The toggle-torque-recoil move, for instance, is designed to free the joints and release the tension being held in the surrounding muscles.

McTimoney practitioners undergo a long training which includes a large commitment to clinical experience. They prefer to work, where possible, in conjuction with doctors. If you are new to the idea of chiropractice, this is a good place to start.

Manual Lymphatic Drainage/

Skin Brushing

Good for: acne and other skin complaints, arthritis, inflammation, sinusitus, burn wounds and boosting the immune system

It sounds more like a plumbing job than a relaxing hands-on therapy – and in a way, it is. Popular on the continent but still relatively new to some countries, including the UK, Manual Lymphatic Drainage (MLD) it is a form of massage designed to stimulate the lymph system to eliminate toxins, waste products, bacteria, excess water and viruses.

Developed in France in the 1930s by the Danish physical therapist Dr E. Vodder, it consists of a serious of manipulations to achieve this stimulation and elimination, and to prevent congestions which can otherwise cause problems, especially skin complaints.

The therapist uses four basic movements: the stationary, circular movement; a pumping action; a rotation technique, and a scooping movement. Once gently stimulated, the tissues are then stroked in the direction the lymph should be flowing towards sites of normal lymphatic drainage. Unlike the blood, the lymph system has no pumps or valves to push it around the body and its organs. Instead, it must rely on movement, which is why a 30-minute walk each day is such a good health tonic.

A simple way to encourage a healthy lymph flow at home is to alternate hot and cold showers, followed by skin brushing with the natural bristles of a long-handled skin brush designed specifically for this purpose and available from good health stores. Always brush with upward and circular motions. The skin will redden but it should not hurt. If you feel discomfort, you are being too vigorous.

The lazy version of Manual Lymphatic Drainage involves the use of leg-length plastic covers which are inflated with a pump and then left to vibrate to stimulate lymph flow as you lie on the treatment couch. Think of those padded wine cooler covers and imagine a larger version covering both your legs. All you have to do is lie back in the beauty salon, think of England and hope that nobody who knows you steps through the door.

The Metamorphic Technique

Meditate: Man's problem today is not only has he lost the way; he's lost the address

Nicolas Bardyaev

If you're lucky enough to stumble across this treatment, you'll wonder how come everyone else seems to know about it but you. There's a lot of secrecy surrounding it, partly because it attracts high fliers who wouldn't want their families or their bosses to know what they're doing, and partly because it's so difficult to explain just what it entails.

The Metamorphic Technique is a relative of reflexology. Both start with the practitioner taking your foot in his or her hands. The similarity, though, stops there. Good metamorphic practitioners see themselves as simply holding the energy while the clients' own life-force gets to work to eliminate the long-held emotional blockages which may be holding someone back from reaching their full potential.

The theory is that traumas (from the moment of conception) are held within the memory of every cell in the body, and that until these memories are released you will be blocked from moving on and fulfilling your life's true purpose.

I like this technique because (1) it gets results and (2) your intellect cannot sabotage the process. It seems to work despite, and not because of, your involvement.

When you arrive for your first hour-long session, you'll be asked to remove your shoes and socks and make yourself comfortable, either in a chair or on a couch. The practitioner will take your foot in his or her hand and begin gently to prod along the outside edge of the foot, following a line that runs from the end of your big toe to the back of your heel, tracing the arch of your foot. This gentle movement follows the spinal reflexes, and this area of the foot is said to represent and reflect the nine, almost ten months you were in your mother's womb.

You are not required to do anything. You can talk, or not, as you please. Lots of men like this technique because it's OK to fall asleep and not speak. The practititioner will work on both feet and then mirror this same action on both of your hands, running from the tip of the index finger along the arch again to the end of the thumb. Finally, attention is turned to your head – for me, this was where the real work started.
During a session you'll probably be aware of energy moving around inside your

body. This can feel like a mild tingling or a rush of heat up the spine. You may sometimes feel nothing; that's fine too. Commonly-reported after-effects, especially after the first few sessions, can include flu-like symptoms (but without the fever), a stomach upset, tearfulness, chronic tiredness or aching limbs.

The number of sessions you need is entirely up to you. Some people go once a week, others once a month. I had weekly sessions for nine months and then stopped. You can go back for 'top-up' sessions when you feel the need.

The changes that may occur will vary between individuals too, but what almost everyone who has experienced this technique agrees is that these changes, when they do come, are always dramatic. I looked in my supermarket trolley one day and realised it was full of vegetables. I realised I couldn't remember when I'd last given in to temptation and had a cigarette or an alcoholic drink. Quite simply, these props no longer featured in my life. I found I couldn't eat meat and I couldn't stand crowds or excessive noise. It was as if, physically, I'd been spring-cleaned. Emotionally, I felt as if I'd shed all the traumas that had been blighting my life and could finally move on.

This technique gets real results but is not for the faint-hearted. Although it appears you do no work, once the life-force gets going again the speed with which you move ahead may leave you feeling dizzy.

Mora Therapy

If you like the idea of playing health detective, this technique will have you hooked. In the hands of the trained practitioner it is a fascinating investigation of what is going on with your body, on every level, at that exact moment.

Described as a form of bio-resonance treatment, Mora Therapy is used to test the body for imbalances, as well as food intolerance and allergies. It can also be used to identify nutritional deficiencies, and to find the correct homoeopathic remedy for you.

An entirely painless form of electroacupuncture, this is another device created by a medically qualified doctor – F. Morrel, MD. Said to be highly effective against headaches, muscular pain and circulatory defects, I was first introduced to it by holistic skin therapists, who use it successfully to treat a wide range of skin disorders but especially eczema, psoriasis, rosacea and acne.

The theory is that the Mora machine, which is no bigger than a shoebox, can pick up electromagnetic waves from your body. It will then manipulate those that have gone awry, by increasing or decreasing their amplitude, before sending them back into the body to effect a cure. Where the detective work comes in is in finding which nutritional or mineral deficiencies may be responsible for disturbing these electromagnetic waves, and which nutritional remedies, in which dosage, will correct them.

A good practitioner will draw on his or her clinical experience, intuition and training in homoeopathy and/or nutrition, plus a detailed knowledge of your medical history to work out what underlies the problem and to prescribe the correct solution. A full assessment can take up to two hours, but there is no discomfort involved since the electrode probes used are applied only to acupressure points on the fingers and toes. You hold one probe in your right hand to form the circuit, the practitioner uses another to test your body's responses.

To me, the big advantage of having this type of investigation, even if nobody can really explain why it should work, is that you can see for yourself how the Mora machine rebalances when certain nutrients or homeopathic remedies are brought into the circuit. Compliance is as big a problem in complementary medicine as it is in orthodox treatment. For me, having seen the practitioner use the Mora machine to work out precisely what I needed and why, I find I feel much more motivated to carry on taking the vitamins, tissue salts or homoepathic remedy that is then prescribed for me.

Phytobiophysics

If I were a flower, I would be a lupin (apparently). I am quite pleased about this because this is one plant that has, despite my worst efforts at a cottage garden, managed to thrive in my borders and so, if nothing else, it (and I) must be pretty hardy.

I was told my flower type by the flower therapist Diana Mossop (who says she is a pansy). She has made a lifelong study of the extraodinary powers of plant essences to produce a fascinating range of flower formulas, which she launched at the end of the 1990s.
Mossop, who was born in Nyasaland in 1947 and who spent the first few years of her life living in the heart of the African bush, was once the youngest captain in the British Army. Her own illness through mercury (dental amalgam)

poisoning and the emotional after-effects of divorce led her back to her family roots in Jersey, where she started working as a beauty therapist.

She says she felt a strong affinity for working with flower essences (see Flower Remedies, page 286), and decided to develop her own, together with a new treatment philosophy. This, in turn, led to establishing The Institute of Phytobiophysics in Jersey, which now trains other practitioners in the use of plant energy to restore balance, harmony and wellness.

If you can choose your favourite colour, then you can treat yourself with one or more of her range of 20 flower formulas. Mossop is not allowed by law to make any medical claims for her products, but one of London's top nutritional consultants told me, independently, that she rates these products very highly and that when she has given the Red Chrysanthemum formula (FF19) to people who have been suffering from severe constipation, they practically skip to the toilet.

According to Mossop, her flower pills, which are beautifully packaged, work on a physical, emotional and spiritual level. Orchid (FF7), for example, is said to work its magic on the ears and to promote fulfillment. Nightshade (FF5) is said to boost immunity and maintain a healthy mouth, including the teeth. Thistle (FF4) works on the head and encourages peaceful sleep and tranquillity.

Mossop has, in fact, tapped into a philosophy that many are calling the medicine of the future - vibrational medicine (see the Medicine Now! chapter) – which is based on the idea that we all vibrate at a specific frequency – which can be matched to a colour or sound, both of which are now used by some practitioners to heal. With these flower formulas and other flower essence ranges, including the Bach Flower Remedies, your vibration is matched to that of a plant, and it is this vibrational energy that is used to treat illness in your body.

The theory is that disease and stress can cause energy blocks which distort the frequency at which, in optimum health, we should be vibrating. Mossop argues that this is the deep level at which her flower formulas work. I gave two of her formulas (Dandelion for detoxifying and White Rose for recovery) to a new dad, who admitted to a terrible hangover after 'wetting the baby's head' a little too enthusiastically. Two hours after feeling so ill that he could not face a glass of water, let alone lunch, he positively bounced into my house and demolished a large bowl of vegetable stew.

Phytoligotherapy (Trace Mineral Therapy with Herbs)

If you ever studied physics or chemistry at school, you will remember the Periodic Table. The names of the elements may not have meant much to you then, but since you are now interested in complementary health, they will become more and more familiar. Try getting by without calcium, for example, crucial for strong bones and teeth. Without it, your skeleton would snap. There is magnesium, the most important mineral for the heart, and iron, without which you would not only become anaemic but tired, weak and even brain-fatigued.
Less well known but equally important to your health and well-being are the so-called trace elements or trace minerals – they may be needed in only miniscule amounts, but they are just as important to your body's healthy

functioning as the 'major' minerals we all know about.

Most of the food we eat is made up of carbon, hydrogen, oxygen and nitrogen. Everything else on your plate can be collectively referred to as the mineral content. There are at least 25 minerals; of these, there are 16 which you must have in your diet. These are used in the skeleton, in the cells and in the body's own fluids. While nutritionists and other food experts can publish useful guidelines recommending a minimum daily intake of the better-known minerals, the fact is that nobody really knows how much of the trace elements you need in your diet to stay healthy. What is known, though, is that without some of them, the better-known minerals will not do their job either.

Iron is one of the biggest nutritional deficiencies, especially in women who, over the course of a month, lose twice as much of this blood-building mineral as men. Only about 8% of your total iron intake ever actually reaches your bloodstream; this figure falls even lower if you are lacking in the trace element copper, which the body needs to better absorb the iron it does get in the diet.

The trace elements include some names you will know and others that will be new to you: manganese, cobalt, iodine, copper, selenium, vanadium, nickel, boron, fluorine, molybdenum, chromium, germanium (see Chapter 2) and zinc. The last is involved in more than 200 different processes in the body, from skin repair to sperm production and immune support.

Copper has cancer-protecting antioxidant properties and is important for the manufacture of collagen to keep the skin elastic and the bones flexible. Iodine is involved with the master thyroid gland, which controls so many other functions.

Chromium, which works to boost the absorption of the energy-fuel glucose by the body's cells, can even help people with diabetes reduce their reliance on insulin.

Intensive farming techniques have stripped the soil of trace elements; this is the main reason so many people are deficient in one or more of these important chemicals. One US study, for example, found that the grass plains in Florida had become so depleted of copper, the cattle were suffering from osteoporosis.

One of the more appealing therapies designed to replenish low levels of the trace elements is *Phytoligotherapy*, which combines minerals with herbs designed to boost their action or absorption further. Also known as Phytoligo Trace Element Therapy, it is not a DIY-technique and is only available through a trained health practitioner.

I first came across it via my homoeopath, who prescribed artichoke with trace elements to stimulate my liver and digestion, and juniper – again, together with trace elements – to cleanse my kidneys and accelerate a spring detox programme.

Think back to that Periodic Table and you will know how, in the wrong doses, trace elements can be toxic to the body. This is one reason I like the Phytoligo range, where the missing trace elements are made available in an active but non-toxic form.

So, how do you know, without visiting an alternative health practitioner, if you need to boost your trace elements? If you are vegetarian, the chances are high that you will be deficient in one or more of the trace elements, since so many of them come from meat and meat products. If you do not eat meat, you may want to investigate supplementing your diet with a good multivitamin including the trace elements.

There is though, some difficulty in accurately assessing levels of any of the minerals in the body, trace or otherwise. Relying on blood tests, for example, can be unhelpful since the body works hard to keep its blood nutrient levels balanced, sometimes at the cost of other systems. This means any deficiency that does show up in the blood is likely to be an extreme one which has already taken its toll elsewhere in the body.

Some researchers have been investigating using hair and fingernail analysis to measure for minerals, including the trace elements. While this may be a useful research tool, there is not a huge body of clinical evidence – certainly not enough to make any claim of an industry standard. These kinds of tests are, however, very good if you are testing for heavy metal toxicity. Otherwise, unless you know what is happening behind the scenes, you may need to take the results with a pinch of salt.

The name may be a mouthful, but in the right hands Phytoligotherapy takes the guesswork out of mineral deficiencies.

What Really Works – Easy Mineral Guide

The Big League

Calcium: present in bones and teeth and needed for blood-clotting, muscle contraction and nerve activity
Sources: milk, cheese, bread, fortified flour, cereals, sea greens, cooked rhubarb, green vegetables

Phosphorous: also in bones and teeth. Essential for energy storage, cell division and reproduction
Sources: dairy products, cereals, meat and meat products

Sodium: found in the body fluids and crucial for maintaining those fluids, muscle contraction and nerve function
Sources: salt, bread, cereals, meat, meat products

Potassium: present in cell fluid, it plays a similar role to sodium
Sources: wide variety of vegetables, meat, milk, fruit and fruit juices

Iron: essential part of haemoglobin – the oxygen-carrying part of the red blood cells
Sources: meat, offal, bread, potatoes, vegetables

Magnesium: present in bone and cell fluids. Needed by many enzymes for chemical reactions in the body and for the absorption of calcium
Sources: milk, bread, cereal products, potatoes, vegetables

Zinc: essential for many enzymes involved in energy production, the reproductive system, the immune system and the formation of proteins
Sources: milk, cheese, meat, meat products, bread flour, cereals, pumpkin seeds

The Little League

Selenium: linked with vitamin E activity and so has antioxidant properties. Now the subject of the first UK clinical trial investigating minerals and cancer protection
Sources: cereals, fish, meat, nuts

Copper: needed for healthy blood; present in many enzymes
Sources: green vegetables, fish, liver

Chromium: involved in the metabolism of glucose, the body's fuel
Sources: liver, cereals, beer, yeast

Iodine: critical component of the thyroid hormones
Sources: seafoods, milk, iodized salt

Manganese: protects against cell damage and heart disease
Sources: tea, cereals, pulses, nuts

Cobalt: builds red blood cells
Sources: liver and other meats

Fluorine: another component of the thyroid hormones
Sources: milk, seafood, iodized salt
Molybdenum: cleanses the body of toxins and plays a role in kickstarting the enzymes which are the catalysts for all biochemical reactions in the body
Sources: kidney, cereals, vegetables

Pilates

Good for: performers, sportsmen and -women, those who are new to exercise, older people who want to build strength and flexibility, pregnant women, new mothers and anyone wanting a flat stomach!

When a dot.com whizzkid who had just signed up a celebrity actress to front his then new complementary health site was asked in a serious television documentary interview what unique medical qualification she brought to the venture, his response was: 'She does Pilates.'

Pilates, pronounced pee-lah-tees, was once the best-kept secret in showbiz. Dancers, actors, musicians and TV presenters, as well as top sportsmen and -women, were among the devoted practitioners of this body conditioning programme which promises to flatten your stomach in just weeks.

The attraction lies in the fact that the exercises are designed to build muscle, tone, flexibility and strength without adding bodybuilder bulk. This is achieved by doing specific slow, controlled movements which avoid any risk of injury. In fact, you are not allowed to move until you are in the right postural position.

It is named after German-born Joseph H. Pilates, who'd been a sickly child but who went on to become a keen sportsman. He moved to the US as young man, having first devised this fitness programme as a prisoner of war in England where, so the story goes, he passed it on to other internees.

In America, the technique – which teaches proper breathing and body alignment

– was taken up with enthusiasm by a number of ballet companies and even a police force or two. Originally called Contrology, it is the perfect regimen for pregnant women and excellent for re-defining your body shape after birth. It promotes relaxation, making it a good antidote to stress, and is popular among people with back problems who have to avoid other forms of exercise.

To get started you will need to find a teacher to learn the basics, some of which you can then practise at home. One of my favourite exercises, which anyone can do at home, consists of rolling your foot over a tennis ball to exercise all the tiny bones in the foot. Many Pilates stretches, though, can only be done in a Pilates studio equipped with special machines designed for these specific movements.

Pilates classes have sprung up in gyms all over the country; in these classes you will concentrate on mat work. A number of these exercises have their roots in yoga, and some positions, like the cat, even have the same name that they have in yoga.

Reflexology

Good for: no good reflexologist will make any medical claims, but reflexology can help alleviate an enormous number of conditions, ranging from post-natal depression to skin disorders, loss of libido or diarrhoea.

It is also an excellent introduction to natural healing and to preventative medicine, especially if you are just looking for something to help you relax, alleviate anxiety and counter stress.

Everyone knows reflexology as the technique where the soles of the feet are massaged, but few people realise it does not have to confine itself to the feet. For those who hate anyone touching this part of their body (and lots of people do), hand reflexology is an excellent alternative. In fact, you can practise reflexology on any part of the body.

With foot reflexology, the idea is that illness stems from a blockage in the way your energy (what the Chinese call *chi*) flows. Although reflexology was practised in ancient China; an even earlier form was also popular in ancient Egypt and was used by indigenous African and Native American peoples to keep healthy.

The technique taught today though, was developed by an American ear, nose and throat doctor called William Fitzgerald. He divided the body into 10 equal, vertical zones that ended in the fingers and toes. Known then as Zone Therapy, this was further refined in the 1930s to produce the version of reflexology that is now so widely used.

Reflexologists are taught that energy channels connect your feet directly to other specific parts of the body. They learn that the left foot represents the left-hand side of the body and that the right foot mirrors the right side.

At your first session, the therapist will take a detailed medical history before examining and massaging your feet. You may be asked to wash your feet before treatment begins and, once you have, they may then be dusted with a coating of talcum powder in preparation for the massage.

The therapist uses his or her thumbs to massage each of the tiny reflex points on the soles of the feet. The heel of the foot, for instance, represents the pelvic area, the pad is linked to the lungs, breast and chest, the bottom of the big toe links to the hormone-controlling pituitary gland and the internal organs connect to the middle of the sole.

By stimulating the relevant reflexes, the therapist is able to improve the circulation of blood to various areas of the body and, it is said, trigger the body's own healing mechanisms. If there is a problem in any particular area, you may experience a sharp but short-lived stabbing pain. The therapist may then spend a little more time on this area, but the general idea is to give the whole body a treatment.

Reiki

Good for: stress, relaxation, headaches, insomnia and general well-being, but attracts more than its share of cranks and wannabe healers

A version of touch therapy where the practitioner heals those parts of the body which he or she senses are weakened, Reiki is a form of massage that originated in Japan.

I have no problem with the technique, but I do have a problem with the notion that anyone can become a practitioner after a couple of weekend courses, and that some people will even call themselves 'Masters' after such limited training.

I have written about this concern before and it prompted a flurry of indignation from angry practitioners, all suggesting I had some personal vendetta against this healing therapy. I don't. I just don't like the idea of inexperienced people getting their hands on the needy, the sick, the vulnerable and the naive.

The idea behind Reiki is that the practitioner can channel the life-force to do the necessary healing. The Japanese word *rei* means 'universal' or 'spiritual'; *ki* means 'life-force'.

People who have tried Reiki report a deep sense of well-being and relaxation at the end of a session, but the first time I came across Reiki, it was at the hands of a beautician who, somewhat arrogantly, did not bother to tell me what she was doing. I could feel heat in the areas where she placed her hands – some people report feeling cold or a tingling sensation as the energy flows – but I was not confident she knew just what she was up to or why. To be treated, you lie, fully-clothed, on a treatment couch.

Although Reiki has its roots in ancient Tibetan Buddhist healing, the form most widely practised today was re-discovered by Dr Mikao Usi, a Japanese theologian working in the late 19th century. It was then brought to the West by a female practitioner called Hawaio Takata in the 1960s.

You can learn to treat yourself, but to do so you must first train to what is called the first degree level. There are three levels or degrees of qualification and you can only train under the guidance of a Reiki Master who will initiate you through an energy attunement.

The Master channels universal life energy to clients, family and friends. The practitioner is then said to act as a conduit for cosmic energy which enters through the top of the head and exits via the hands.

There is much competition surrounding the pedigree of a Master who tunes any particular practitioner. Make sure, if you seek out this treatment or training, you check out the credentials of those planning to interact with you. True energy healing requires pure channels, and not everyone claiming to be a Reiki practitioner is as 'pure' as you might wish them to be.

Shiatsu

Good for: chronic conditions including back pain, insomnia, migraine, digestive disorders, arthritis, asthma and back pain; it also encourages rest and relaxation

Sometimes described as acupuncture without the needles, Shiatsu is a Japanese form of massage which, like acupuncture, works to rebalance the life-force or *chi*. The word itself means 'finger pressure', but a Shiatsu therapist is just as likely to use his or her palms, knuckles, elbows, knees and, in some cases, even their feet if that is what is required to remove energy blockages and get the chi flowing.

Shiatsu works on the principle that all disease is the result of a disturbance in the flow of chi (*ki* in Japanese), through the body. Your energy may be depleted (*kyo*), blocked, or over-active (*jitsu*); the theory is that any disturbance manifests itself on the surface of the body at points which are called *tsubos*.

There are over 600 of these points, which the therapist will manipulate to promote and re-establish well-being. They may stretch your limbs and even move the position of your entire body to get to the root of the problem.

You keep your clothes on throughout a Shiatsu massage, so wear something loose and comfortable. The practitioner will take a full medical history and you will then lie on a mat or futon for the massage itself. Some of the points that are manipulated may feel a little bit sore, but this will pass and you will emerge feeling refreshed and revitalised.

I once had a Shiatsu face massage which was so gentle I did not believe any good could have come of it. I was so disappointed, I considered asking for my money back. Two days later, I walked into work and was stopped en route to my desk by every other 30-something female colleague, all of whom wanted to know what I had done to my face. I looked in the mirror and saw what they were seeing. It was as if the years had rolled back; my skin looked fresh and rejuvenated, and many of the more ageing face lines had faded or gone. Of course the effect was only temporary, but it was wonderful to get so many compliments over the following week.

If you are planning to try this massage, do not eat for two hours before a session. If you think you may be pregnant, tell the therapist – he or she will then avoid stimulating certain points. A Shiatsu massage is contraindicated if you have chronic high blood pressure, a blood-borne cancer, any history of brain haemorrhage, any contagious disease or a high fever.

One of the things I like best about this type of massage is that it must be one of the few disciplines where one of the ruling bodies, The Shiatsu Society, can put its hand on its collective heart and report, truthfully, that since the 1970s, when Shiatsu was first introduced to the West, it has never had a single complaint from a dissatisfied customer.

Spiritual Healing

The laying on of hands is as old as the Bible, but then a lot of the practices we now consider New Agey have their roots in far older religious and healing traditions.

The theory with spiritual healing is that healing energy is all around us and so all the spiritual healer does, is act as a channel or conduit to target that energy to the person (and even the organ or body part) that needs it. Some healers say this energy comes directly from God. Others tell me it is a kind of cosmic, universal healing force which we can all tap into once we know how.

Most people find their way to this type of healing as a last resort, but far from being seen as fringe or wacky, it is actually the most extensive therapeutic system outside orthodox, mainstream medicine.

If the idea that someone can lay their hands on or close to you and heal you is far too way out for you, you are going to struggle even more with the notion of absent healing. I have never sought this kind of healing for myself, but then I have never felt the need to. If I found myself with a chronic or painful condition from which I was getting no relief, this would probably be one of my first ports of call.

I have witnessed this same kind of healing performed on animals and, as we all know, they cannot be responding to an imaginary effect. I have also become increasingly aware that many complementary health practitioners who do not call themselves healers are, in fact, working in this way, whether they know it or not. You can feel the heat when their hands come near you, and I am certain that this is a skill we could all develop if we felt so inclined.

In the UK, hospital patients are now legally permitted to request a spiritual healer to come onto the wards, and since the majority of the healers I have met are lovely, well-meaning people, this can only be a good thing. Better still, most of the good healers who know what they are doing and who treat their abilities as a special gift say it doesn't matter whether you believe it or not since, as long as their intentions are right, it will work.

What is clear is that healing has its roots in cultures that had no doctors or high-tech equipment to save lives. Western healers may not work with an eagle feather or dance themselves into a shamanic trance, but what they are doing is not so very different from the work of the tribal medicine men and women in the indigenous tribes. If, like the shamans, you believe a great deal of sickness and disease has its roots in a spiritual malaise, then the idea of spiritual healing makes good sense.

Watsu

Good for: stress, mobility, insomnia, boosting energy levels and learning to let go

Watsu is Shiatsu in the water and, according to practitioners, is a very unthreatening way to release both physical and especially emotional tensions that you may have been holding on to for years.
Devised by Harold Dull, director of the School of Shiatsu and Massage in Harbin Hot Springs, California, the idea is that because the body is supported in water, it is more relaxed and therefore more responsive to the Shiatsu touch.

Watsu sessions take place in a hydrotherapy pool where the water is heated to body temperature to recreate the warmth of the protective amniotic fluid that we float in during gestation. To benefit, you will need to get over the odd feeling of someone else handling your body while you close your eyes and try to trust them enough to truly let go.

The technique concentrates on freeing up the spine. The support of the water allows the therapist to move your spine in ways that are just not possible on land, and so some say the benefits are even greater than with normal Shiatsu.

The practitioner will take your body through a series of moves with apt-sounding names like The Dolphin or The Cradle. The physical impact is usually a feeling of being less rigid in your body. The emotional reaction can be as extreme as bursting into tears, shaking or simply laughing. Whatever way your body releases, it will benefit from the session.

I like Watsu since it is non-threatening and perfect for those who may not normally feel comfortable with such intimate contact, especially children who have suffered any form of abuse and subsequently keep their physical distance from others.

The movement of the water against the body also works to stimulate the lymphatic system, and so it is also a good therapy for encouraging the release of toxins and waste products. You may feel dehydrated after a session, so make sure you rehydrate by drinking plenty of pure water.

Zero Balancing

*Our deepest nature is held in bone, and when you touch
someone this way, they certainly know about it.*

Dr Fritz Smith, creator of Zero Balancing

Good for: this gentle but powerful technique will change your life, for the
better, in ways you can only guess at right now

This potent but little-known therapy is another of those well-kept healing
secrets. Described as massage with your clothes on, therapy without the talk and
meditation without the mantra, it goes right to the heart of healing by bringing
your energy and your physical body into balance.

It has only been around for 20 years and is, according to its founder, US
physician and osteopath Dr Fritz Smith, the first healing technique to work on
the mind and body by truly integrating the Eastern concept of energy flow with
a Western understanding of body structure.

To explain this, Smith describes a sail boat being powered by the wind. Think of
the sail as the structure (your skeleton) and the wind as the energy. Energy,
argues Dr Smith, is just like the physical body. It has its own anatomy,
physiology and pathology. This is clearly understood in the East but is a
relatively new concept for many Western healers.

The name Zero Balancing is something of a misnomer, since it doesn't tell you
the first thing about this therapy. It was, apparently, coined when a client
jumped off the couch after a session and said: 'I feel fantastic, I feel zero
balanced.'

Yes, you do lie on a couch, but only after an assessment of the current state of your energy field and your skeletal flexibility. For this, you sit on the edge of the couch and allow your pelvis to be rocked from side to side and your arms to be rotated in their sockets. You then lie down and do nothing for the 40 minutes an average session will last.

The ZB practitioner has been trained to recognise energy pathways clearly mapped out by Dr Smith, and so your session will always follow the same pattern. The therapist uses fulcrums or 'pivotal points' which they themselves create in your body using the pressure of their fingertips. They believe this brings your energy and structure into a balanced relationship and helps them hold it there for a few seconds.

Zero balancing again reminds me of The Bowen Technique (see page 275), which applies a similar self-healing principle and which those who suffer from muscular-skeletal and joint problems swear by. Zero balancing, though, takes the whole concept one step further by bringing in a spiritual quality that can make your session more like a meditation.

Zero Balancers (or Zee-Bee-ers, as they call themselves) are highly trained. Most have a bodywork background such as massage or osteopathy; you should immediately feel you are being worked on by someone who knows their way around the body and who knows exactly what they are doing. When the practitioner creates the fulcrum that brings together your energy and structure in a perfect balance, you feel a deep but painless pressure at that point.

Whatever state you are in when you first get onto the couch, you can expect to jump off again feeling relaxed, lighter in your body, beautifully stretched out and quieter. You will though feel differently both during and after each individual session. Sometimes you may float off with a feeling of deep contentment and bliss. You may, when you step down, realise your legs feel like jelly and that your head is still reeling from the deep meditation. You may feel a release either during or after a treatment, and if you feel overwhelmed by the urge to cry, then do. Your therapist will not be surprised. At the end of a session, whatever your reaction, take your time to come back. Have a biscuit and a herbal tea to remind your body this is the dimension it belongs to.

Zero Balancing can relieve muscular-skeletal problems and help clear other blockages and emotional or spiritual issues. It helped me clear a path in my life for the non-work matters I considered important but was guilty of neglecting, and gave me a sense of my own innate strength and ability to heal myself. You will certainly, at least for a few hours after a session, walk taller both literally and metaphorically, and you may feel yourself more firmly in and of the world.

It would be all too easy to become addicted to the blissful feelings you often experience both during and after ZB but unless you are dealing with a specific problem, such as back pain or headaches, then you probably only need a session once every three weeks to help you stay both connected and in balance.

 **SoulWorks**

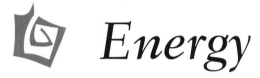 # Energy

Bioenergetics – Your Secret Weapon

They say that 50 is the new 30, but that's no consolation when you are so tired, stressed and run ragged by the demands of your daily life you feel twice as old as your true biological age. Seeing glamorous photographs of supposedly inspirational role models is only going to make you feel worse. None of us – not even those airbrushed supermodels – can truly stop the biological clock, but that is not what counts. What really matters is not how old you are but how you feel when you wake up in the morning.

Cosmetic surgery, anti-wrinkle potions and anti-ageing hormone pills may help you win the battle against the march of time for a few years, but if you want to work with your body to rejuvenate your cells and keep your insides as young as you would like them to be, you need to get down to some basic biochemistry and get to grips with the new and fascinating science of Bioenergetics. This is going to be the secret weapon that helps you cheat the ageing process and gives you back the kind of energy stores you took for granted when you were young.

Believe me, once you have grasped the basics you will not only be glad you have taken the time to learn how to boost your energy, you will also start to feel so much better that your friends will be snooping around your bathroom cupboards trying to find the secret elixir that has put a sparkle back into your eyes, a glossy sheen on your hair, a youthful glow to your skin and more than a spring in your step.

If there is one complaint that overshadows every other 21st-century health niggle, it is that feeling of being tired and having no real energy. You know several cups of coffee or a chocolate bar will rev the engine and get you going in the short term, but you also know that these are nothing more than a quick fix and that, unless you can replenish your energy stores at a deeper level, you are on a hiding to nothing.

There is nothing more depressing than thinking back to your childhood and remembering how you had more zip than you (or your frazzled parents) could handle. Where did it all go? Wouldn't it be amazing to wake up every morning feeling re-energised and ready to face another busy day, knowing you will take everything in your stride and still have enough energy left over to do some of those things you keep promising yourself you'll do – like working out at the gym or taking your partner out for a night on the town?

There are supplements and herbs that can re-energise a tired body and help you wake up feeling enthused and refreshed every day, but they cannot work miracles on their own. You need to give them a helping hand. That means making a commitment to looking after yourself in every sense of the word. You will need to make sure you are, for the most part, eating the right kinds of health-promoting foods that will keep your cells nourished and fuelled. You will need to try and avoid the obvious toxins and pollutants that are prematurely ageing (cigarettes, too much alcohol and too many high-fat, high-sugar take-outs), and you are going to have to make a point of taking enough time out to give tired cells a chance to repair and recuperate.

You will also have to learn how to recognise the warning signs of a body slowing down, long before it crashes through exhaustion. This means learning to listen to your body's own wisdom about just how far and how long you can push it. For example, we all thrive and perform well when under a moderate amount of short-lived stress and pressure, but we begin to wipe ourselves out (and, in the process, accelerate premature ageing) when we allow stress to control our lives. The secret to healthy living is to recognise the warning signs and learn when your body has had enough.

Why Stress Is the No. 1 Energy-depleting Enemy

I have to admit, when I was younger and had enough energy to waste most of it burning the candle at both ends, I thought stress was all in the mind. It seemed a too-convenient label for far too many conditions, a great way of blaming the patient for whatever was wrong with them and the perfect cop-out for the workplace 'wimps' who could not take the pace or hack it any more.

When the time came for me to learn the error of my own ways, it was nothing short of a slap around the face.

I was juggling a number of work and domestic pressures. Nothing that I would not have been able to handle individually but, coming all together, it was just too much. The first tell-tale sign was the fact that I started feeling miserable. It was the end of a long British winter and I would normally have been feeling uplifted by the first shoots of spring, but I felt as if there was nothing to look forward to; all that existed were the grinding demands of that particular day. I would drag myself out of bed to sit at my computer, sometimes for 10 hours at a time, trying to juggle all my writing deadlines and wondering why I was so miserable. I had escape fantasies which always involved a kind of sneaking away. I imagined packing the smallest suitcase, taking the smaller car and even the smallest of my two dogs and just disappearing into the night. I was on the verge of tears all the time and started to think my entire existence was pointless. It didn't matter how hard I worked or how rigidly I stuck to my schedule, the days seemed to keep getting shorter and I was getting less and less done.

These horrible feelings went on for two months. I was shocked by how difficult it was to ask anyone for help, since I felt my problems, especially the horrendous work deadlines, were self-inflicted. I wrote my first book, *The Vitality Cookbook*, working on and testing over 100 recipes with the French-trained chef Erick Muzard, in just two months to meet the publishers' unreasonable deadlines. (I later learned nobody ever meets the deadline and, in any event, they edited another book before mine, which meant it sat gathering dust for three months!)

I still shudder when I think back to how sick I was on the way to becoming. I could not sleep, I began to crave junk food and I felt as though I was on the verge of a panic attack all the time. I was so caught up in this downward spiral I did not even realise what was going on until I began to write about stress for my book and saw all my own symptoms, in black and white, staring back at me.

I had thought I was depressed and heading for a work-related breakdown. In fact, I was exhausted, worn out by the prolonged stress of endless deadlines. Tiredness and an energy crisis, nothing else, were causing my depression.

The events most likely to trigger unhealthy stress are job pressures, family arguments, financial worries and deadlines, but anything that upsets the normal equilibrium can cause of number of biological – and very real – changes, that typify stress and which are known collectively as General Adaptation Syndrome (GAS).

There are three distinct phases to GAS. You will, if you are short of energy, recognise all three. In the first phase, most of your energy is spent worrying that you cannot do everything you think you should be doing. In phase II, the mind is still willing but the body is beginning to put the brakes on. The last phase is the one you really want to avoid, since this is the one where you collapse in an exhausted heap and fall sick.

All three of these phases are controlled by the adrenal glands, which regulate hormone levels and which can themselves become exhausted. They pump out a hormone called cortisol which helps the brain stay alert. In good health, levels are higher in the morning when we need the brain to function at its best, and then drop towards the evening when we want to slow down. When the body is suffering from prolonged stress, the adrenals keep the cortisol levels too high, making you hyperalert day and night. The two biggest signs of this type of adrenal stress are sweating for no apparent reason, especially at night, and waking up in the early hours of the morning too tired to get up but unable to get back to sleep.

If you have reached the point of adrenal exhaustion, you will know it. You will have that panicky stressed-out feeling I have described and it will be taking its toll on your looks and your insides. Your skin may erupt, your hair will become lank and your nails may start splitting. Your digestion will become disrupted and your immune system will be under pressure. Your heart rate speeds up to prepare you for a 'flight' response; you may even have a panic attack.

While the first phase of GAS is relatively short lived, the second (or resistance) phase, which allows you to carry on fighting the stress, can go on and on. You will get a temporary increase in energy to help you do this, and even your blood pressure will go up to keep you alert, but the long-term price is the exhaustion you want to avoid.

Younger bodies are programmed to dispose of stress hormones and return to normal quickly, but for adults who are less active and who have mainly sedentary lifestyles, there is nowhere for these hormones, which can even damage other organs, to go. Too much stress at any age is a bad thing, but the older you get the greater the toll, especially on your energy reserves. Too much stress can also dampen down the immune system, leaving you more prone to infections and other diseases.

Make Friends with Your Mitochondria

To avoid this kind of damaging, stress-related exhaustion, you need to make sure your body has enough energy and more. Bioenergetics shows us how we can do this, by concentrating on the cellular structures where energy is made – the mitochondria.

Known as the powerhouses of the cells, the mitochondria can only be seen under the microscope, which reveals that they are very similar in structure to cells. They have an outer membrane and an inner one. The latter folds in on itself to create shelf-like structures called *cristae*. This is where the real action takes place because this is where your energy is made.

Each mitochondrion produces a substance called adenosine triphosphate, (ATP) which carries the body's fuel reserves. This is the fuel that powers everything that happens in your mind and body, every thought, every step, every heartbeat. You will find between 500 and 2,000 mitochondria in any single cell, with the highest concentrations in those organs that work the hardest – the brain, the heart and the kidneys. They are not present in red blood cells (although they are needed to make these cells) or in the lens of the eye. Otherwise, you find them in every single cell of every animal, plant and organism.

When you are young and have bags of energy, your mitochondria are fit, and healthy and working at optimum output for you, but as you age, so do the mitochondria. They lose their shape and structure, can become hardened and calcified and produce less and less ATP. Also, since mitochondria need energy to make energy, you can see how, as you get older, low energy becomes a significant problem.

This age-related damage to the energy-producing mitochondria, usually caused by normal wear and tear, is now believed to hold the true and most exciting key to controlling the biological clock and slowing down the ageing process.

While most people know each cell in the body has a nucleus with genetic material which tells it what kind of cell it is going to be and what it is going to do, not many people realise that the mitochondria have their own genetic material too. And, according to bioenergetic researchers, it is this genetic material which determines how well and how quickly you are ageing and how strong your energy stores are.

Several studies have now shown more mitochondrial DNA damage in diseased hearts than in healthy ones. In other research, scientists reported that the mitochondrial DNA in the muscles of much older people was not simply damaged, much of it had completely disappeared. Further research is needed, but you do not need to be a rocket scientist to work out that if there is no DNA telling the mitochondria to make energy to power the cells of the muscle tissue, then there is not much hope for that muscle or its elderly owner.

How to Keep Your Mitochondria Healthy

I am a firm believer in preventative health care, but have only ever once come across a simple health programme that made such incredible good sense that, before they knew it, I had my husband, my siblings and my friends all following it and was buying the relevant supplements in bulk.

Dr Erika Schwartz's bioenergetic programme, which promises to take you from Tired to Terrific in just 10 days, is the only plan I have come across which goes straight to the heart of the problem by targeting and supporting the all-important energy-producing mitochondria. And it could not be simpler.

A former ER doctor with a busy suburban practice in New York, Schwartz has devised an Energy Pack programme which has revolutionised the lives of hundreds of tired and worn-out patients. Her excellent book, *Natural Energy – From Tired to Terrific in 10 Days* has all the details (see Bibliography), but in essence her programme revolves around just two supplements: **Carnitine**, which she calls 'The Capsule of Youth' and **Coenzyme Q10**, which she tags 'The Energiser'.

What her programme does is combine these two supplements which are good on their own but unbelievable when you take them together, to boost your energy. This is because carnitine, which is an amino acid produced naturally in the brain, heart and kidneys, but which the body produces less of with increasing age, actually transports fatty acids across the mitchondrial membrane to be made into energy. Coenzyme Q10 is found in every cell where it plays an important role in energy production. It is also a powerful antioxidant. If you lack either one, your energy levels will not be as good as they could be. Together, they will have you revved up and raring to go.

We have already talked about how damage to the DNA of the mitchondria can cause ageing and disease. This is because of something called free radicals. Whenever there is a chemical reaction in the body, including the production of energy, unstable waste molecules are formed. If they are not mopped up, they can seriously damage cells. Carnitine helps remove waste products. Coenzyme Q10, because of its antioxidant action, mops up those left behind.

Carnitine controls stress (which you will remember adversely affects energy levels) by re-regulating the stress hormone, cortisol. It also boosts levels of cytochrome C oxidase, an enzyme needed for energy production, levels of which are 30% lower in older animals than in younger ones. Coenzyme Q10 is often low in those suffering from heart disease; in animal studies it has been shown to fortify the hearts of older rats so that they recover from stress at the same rate as the hearts of younger animals. Even better, both supplements are completely safe, with no side-effects, no contra-indications and, unlike other more restricted substances, including the hormone-replenishing DHEA, are freely available over the counter.

So, how do you know if you really need them?

There are seven easy-to-spot signs of what Dr Schwartz calls an Energy Crisis. If, for instance, your mind is saying 'do it now' but your body is saying 'it can wait until later', you may be on the way to an energy drain. Waking up feeling more tired than when you went to sleep is another sign, as is wishing you could have an afternoon nap.

If your brain feels foggy all the time, if you're eating too much to try and get an instant energy 'hit' and if you're feeling stressed out and depressed, then it is time to boost your energy. If going to sleep is a million times more exciting than the idea of sex, you may also need to give your mitochondria a helping hand.

You can adjust the dosage of carnitine and coenzyme Q10 to reflect just how wiped out you feel, but to start off, Dr Schwartz recommends taking 500mg of carnitine and 30mg of CoQ10 twice a day, with breakfast and with lunch.

How to Ward Off An Energy Crisis

Whenever I feel an energy crisis heading my way I also include magnesium, which is another part of the chemical reaction that produces ATP. If you supplement magnesium you also need to take calcium, since taking one will affect levels of the other. The correct ratio is 2:1 in favour of the calcium, so if you take 400mg of magnesium make sure you are taking 800mg of calcium.

With extra stress in your life, step up the carnitine to 3,000 mg and increase the Coenzyme Q10 to 90mg a day. Also take 1,000mg of evening primrose oil to make sure there are enough of the right fatty acids in your diet for carnitine to transport into the energy-producing mitochondria.

My body seems to respond to stress, pressure and tiredness by getting fixated on chocolate bars, biscuits and other non-healthy but instant energy hits. I know myself well enough now to recognise this sign of fluctuating blood sugar levels, which have such a powerful impact on mood. You can avoid these swings by taking another amino acid called L-glutamine. This works to stabilise blood sugars.

Other Natural Energy Boosters

Tired adrenal glands are one of the first signs of flagging energy levels. The herb Ginkgo biloba, which boosts circulation, can help revive vitality.

All types of ginseng can help keep tiredness at bay, but for frazzled nerves, Siberian ginseng is best.

To keep on good form, make a point of drinking mineral-rich herbal teas. Nettle is excellent and will also help keep the liver decongested.

The B-vitamins are known as nature's own stress busters. They work best when taken together, so make sure you take a good vitamin B complex supplement daily.

The thyroid controls many of the body's functions, including energy production, the metabolism of sugars and fats, your growth rate, the conversion of vitamin A into betacarotene, your heart rate, your blood pressure, your rate of breathing, mental alertness and libido. Thyroid-supporting herbs include kelp, horsetail, watercress, garlic and spirulina. Green tea will also keep the thyroid healthy.

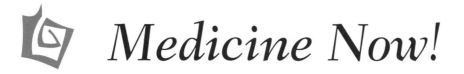

Medicine Now!

Energy is the bridge that connects our physical, emotional and spiritual lives. To work with a person's energy is to touch that person's mind, as well as their body

Donna Eden (USA), Founder of Energy Kinesiology

Biostimulation – Back to the Future

The healthy body is designed to heal itself and Biostimulation is the new name given to those treatments designed to encourage the body to do just that. They range from the different types of Photobiology or Light medicine to the use of

Magnetic Therapy, and work on the principle that if you can trigger a cell to heal itself, you can prevent sickness without resorting to drugs or surgery.

This is not something you are likely to learn from a family physician or any other health practitioner who has been trained and steeped in the drug-led, surgically biased and antibiotic-driven culture of modern medicine which has dominated in the West for the past 75 years, but it is something your ancestors knew intuitively. They did not have the technology or the scientific explanation for why, for example, something that sounds as whacky as light therapy or the stimulation of acupressure points with magnets worked, but they had plenty of empirical evidence. Today, we can claim both.

Light Therapy

Photobiology
Light medicine is being hailed as the medicine of the future, but has, of course, been around for thousands of years. The ancient Greeks, Romans and Egyptians all understood the power of light therapy and recognised its potent healing action on the body, mind and spirit.

Almost a century ago, the father of phototherapy, a Danish physician called Dr Neils Finsen, won the Nobel Prize for medicine for his research into the clinical application of light therapy. He specialised in treating skin tuberculous (lupus) with light therapy and, throughout the 1930s, the idea of using light to help the body heal itself was a popular and widely-accepted treatment option.

Then, as now, it was hailed as the medicine of the future. The UK's prestigious Medical Research Council (MRC) even established a committee on sunlight and another on the health benefits of light, especially for urban dwellers.

Light therapy fell out of favour, however, thanks to the massive shift towards drug-based medicine prompted by the arrival of antibiotics. By the 1950s, it was seen as too whacky and fringe to merit any serious medical attention. For those of us born after this period, it is just as if the heyday of light medicine had never existed, and it is only now being given fair consideration again as a truly holistic tool to encourage the body's own impressive self-healing mechanisms.

Light medicine practitioners take great pains to stress that light itself cannot cure anything. What it does, they argue, is trigger the body to do the job it was designed to do. New research into photobiology suggests that it does have a future, and not just for the treatment of chronic conditions or as a last resort for the desperate patient.

The documented benefits of light therapy include stimulating cellular regeneration, activating the production of adenosine triphosphate (ATP), and triggering the development of new blood vessels. There is also a new technique which, combined with the use of light-sensitising drugs, has been shown in early trials to kill off malignant cancer cells.

The growing acceptance of seasonal affective disorder (SAD), which affects up to 10% of the population in winter and the fact that it can be treated with the use of light boxes has helped overcome some of the deeply ingrained prejudice against light therapy. NASA's acceptance that its astronauts faced serious light-related performance problems which had to be overcome in space has also given the field more credibility and helped to bring light medicine out of the twilight. That said, there are currently several different variations on the theme, some of which are more accepted by the mainsteam than others.

Horse vets and top sportsmen and -women, for example, have long been familiar with the use of light emitting dioxides (LEDs) to accelerate the rate at which a wound or injury heals. It has been shown to halve the normal rate of wound-healing and to reduce the resulting scar size by 50%. It is also used to treat skin problems, chronic pain and autoimmune diseases. The ultra-violet treatment of chronic skin conditions such as acne and psoriasis is now commonplace, and there is growing interest in the use of low levels of soft laser therapy to biostimulate deep bruise- and wound-healing and to heal burns. This treatment depends on the use of red light, which has the longest, deepest-penetrating wavelength.

Photodynamic Therapy (PDT), used in combination with light-sensitising drugs, is the new and exciting light therapy technique which holds some promise for the treatment of cancers. It also uses red light. It is not biostimulatory and so, instead of boosting the immune system, it works to destroy malignant cells. The only recorded side-effect is a fortnight of increased photosensitivity. It does not interfere with other cancer therapies and, if need be, the treatment can be repeated.

PDT is the brainchild of American research chemist Dr Thomas Dougherty. He worked with substances called porphyrins which are a light-sensitising extract of haemoglobin. What he found was that if you injected these intravenously, the porphyrins would flood the patient's whole body and then fade from everywhere but the malignant cells. He discovered UV light would then make those cells fluorescent, and that if you then shone a red light on them, they instantly began to die.

Until now, one of the drawbacks was that because the light had a short reach, it could not penetrate either larger cancer tumours or deep-seated ones, but British scientists at the Centre for Photobiology and Photodynamic Therapy in Leeds have overcome this problem with a technique called interstitial PDT. Here, two or three fibre optics are inserted all the way into the cancer tumour to enable the light dose to be administered right on target. Still not approved in the UK, this technique has had impressive results in research trials with a variety of cancers, including lung cancer.

VIP Light Therapy

This is the other big breakthrough in the brave new world of light medicine. The VIP stands for Visible, Incoherent and Polarised. Here, the light treatment uses wavelengths of between 400 and 2,000 nanometers (nm), which is very similar to the full spectrum produced by natural sunlight – with the exception of the more harmful UV section.

The idea, according to practitioners, is that, just as different vitamins and minerals have different effects on the body, so do different wavelengths of light.

VIP light therapy emerged out of the low-level soft laser technique when scientists decided to investigate how light from lasers affects the biology of the cell. What they found was that the polarisation of light regulates cell membrane activity. Every cell in the body is contained within a membrane, which acts as the mediator between the inner and outer world of the cell. The effect of VIP light on this membrane has now been shown to have an impact on the inside of the cell and its workings.

Russian research carried out by Professor Kira Samilova over the past two decades has shown how VIP light has a gentle, stimulatory effect on the blood flowing through the area being treated, to create something called *photomodulation* – the term used to describe how natural light can boost the immune response of the blood, as well as increase blood supply and energy to every cell. In other words, there is an overall healing effect.

The technique has been used successfully to treat severe second-degree burns, psoriasis, acne, eczema and leg ulcers. It can reduce the appearance of wrinkles and crow's feet, and has even been effective against cellulite.

Even more extraordinary, using VIP light therapy to heal, for example, an ulcer on a patient's leg will also heal the eczema rash on their arm. This has been demonstrated again and again in patients treated with VIP light, and shows how this photomodulated blood carries all its health-giving benefits to all parts of the body for self-healing.

In Russia, where light medicine is taken more seriously, Professor Samilova and her team at the Russian Academy of Sciences in St Petersburg have treated all manner of diseases with UV light. The technique they employ is to irradiate between 1 and 2% of the patient's blood, and to then re-infuse it.

The effect, says the Professor, is instantaneous. The whole of the blood supply changes for the better, to show an improved immune response. This technique is not used as a stand-alone treatment but has proved beneficial in supporting conventional cancer therapies, especially chemotherapy and radiation. The idea is to use light therapy to help restore the body's battered immune system.

If you still think light medicine is for crazies and has no role to play in your own well-being, consider this: In experiments which measure people's response to full-spectrum white light and to the light from a standard fluorescent strip (which, although it looks white, has three or four colours missing), stress-type levels of cortisol and another hormone called adrenocorticotrophic (ACTH) were found in the blood of those subjected to the artificial lighting and not in the group exposed to the full-spectrum white light. Scientists now suggest that artificial lighting could, for example, be to blame for the agitated behaviour of children stuck for long hours under strip lighting in school classrooms. (For more on the importance of natural daylight, read the Sunlight chapter beginning on page 44.)

Colour Therapy

Technically, it is illegal to publish anything in America concerning colour therapy, but many practitioners calling themselves colour puncturists use different colours in strobe light therapy to treat a range of emotional problems. These practitioners work according to the theory that different colours, with their different wavelengths, evoke different emotional and physical responses. A small machine called a Photron is used during this treatment. It emits a gentle flickering coloured strobe which is shone directly into the patient's eyes.

Calming colours – blue and green, for example, are used to treat more recent traumas. More stimulating hues, such as yellow and orange, are used when the problem is a deep-seated psychological block caused by, say, a childhood trauma or other upsetting event that took place a long time ago.

Colour therapy is said to work by affecting the autonomic nervous system. In America, it is used to treat an enormous range of conditions including depression, anxiety, learning problems, dyslexia, problems with poor muscle co-ordination and obsessive compulsive disorders (OCDs). There are still only a limited number of practitioners in Europe where the technique has yet to win any serious medical credibility. That does not mean it will not work for you, it just means your doctor won't believe it!

Biomagnetism

Biomagnetism is another new name for another old and well-established therapy, now regaining mainstream credibility. To accept that biomagnetism has any role in modern healing at all, though, you first have to accept that all living creatures are surrounded by an electromagnetic field (EMF) which can be measured.

Thousands of experiments since the 1930s have proved this to be the case, but what is less well known is that this field is primary and the physical body is secondary. What this means is that changes in the electromagnetic field happen first and are then later followed by changes that you can monitor and see in the physical body. The work of scientist Dr Robert Becker was instrumental in proving this hard-to-grasp concept. He showed that by applying controlled electrical currents which modified these fields, he could, for example, partially regenerate missing limbs in rats.

Other scientists have since shown how manipulating this field can cause and suppress other physical changes, including the stimulation of cancer. These changes do not have to be dramatic, and in fact the strength of the fields used to bring about the changes are usually much lower than the strength of those background electromagnetic fields we are subjected to every day in our offices and homes.

Computers, VDUs, artificial lighting and other office equipment all generate electromagnetic fields and, according to some researchers, people working in such fields are at a much higher risk of cancer and leukaemia than those working in other environments.

This is not intended to scare you, but I do want you to stop and think about this. In one study published by the *American Journal of Industrial Medicine*, scientists monitored 1,583 pregnant women and found that those who spent more than 20 hours a week working at a computer had an 80% higher risk of miscarriage than women who worked away from computers.

Tests carried out by the World Health Organization have also shown how spending just four hours in front the computer screen has an adverse effect on the body's ability to produce adrenalin to cope with stress.

Human testicle cells exposed to the radiation from a computer screen for 24 hours had a 300% increase in mortality.

This kind of 'background radiation' is now being blamed for a number of worrying and increasingly common symptoms, including hormonal disturbances, loss of libido and chronic tiredness.

New thinking on human ageing suggests that the body is not designed to age at all but to go on repairing itself. What goes wrong is the accumulation of a series of malfunctions which prevent this self-healing. EMF fields in the home and workplace are now thought to play a role in this process too.

In ideal conditions, the body is more than able to heal itself. Each cell, for example, is bathed in a fluid from which it takes its nutrients and into which it dumps its waste products. For the cells to stay healthy, this must be an ongoing process and the toxic waste must be removed straight away. For this to happen, both the blood and lymph circulation must be free-flowing and unobstructed.

Since most disease is the result of either toxicity or a deficiency, then any treatment which can maintain this healthy flow of blood and lymphatic drainage is going to benefit your overall health.

This is where Biomagnetism comes in. Once again this is an old therapeutic tool masquerading as something new. Man has been using magnets for healing for centuries. The difference is, he now knows why they work.

The magnets themselves do not heal. What they do is create an environment in the body that encourages self-healing. Think of it as being like acupuncture without the needles.

In Japan, where magnotherapeutic devices already include a system that incorporates magnets into the mattress and pillows of a patient's bedding, researchers have discovered that within just 15 minutes, every single acupressure point on the body of anyone sleeping in this environment has become perfectly balanced. Also, the longer someone sleeps in this system, the more quickly the body can rebalance itself.

A magnetic field enhances both the blood and lymphatic circulation. Users of the magnetic mattress, for example, report both increased warmth in their extremities and a decrease in muscles aches and joint pains. Not surprisingly, in Japan therapeutic magnets are now licensed as medical devices.

For those who fear the hair-thin needles of acupunture, magnets are an excellent alternative. In Russia, doctors routinely use biomagnetism to accelerate wound-healing after surgery and to strengthen and mend bones. Dentists are now learning how magnets can help in pain relief, and in Germany scientists have shown how, in the right hands, magnetic foils can be used to virtually heal unsightly scar tissue.

Magnet therapy uses flexible, rubberized and permanently charged magnetic pads which can be cut into any number of different shapes. These are then attached to an injury site or acupuncture point using athletic tape. With osteoporosis, magnets have been shown to help the body generate new bone growth. This is biostimulation at its best. In further clinical trials of more than 11,000 patients complaining of muscle spasm in the shoulder and neck region, Japanese doctors were able to free 90% of patients from any kind of pain using magnetic pads.

The Future

Nothing can beat conventional medicine in a crisis, and when it comes to acute illness, high-tech medicine is, quite rightly, in the front line. That does not mean, though, that we should turn our backs on techniques that have worked for thousands of years. The idea of an energy system with its own anatomy and physiology may still make Western doctors nervous, but just because something is unfamiliar to us, does not mean it does not work.

True holistic healing means choosing the best healthcare options from every discipline or practice and using it to get 100% better and well again. It does not mean refusing life-saving drugs if you need them, or turning down emergency surgery. It may, though, mean thinking twice about so-called routine operations for conditions that can be managed by less intrusive techniques, including, perhaps, phototherapy or biostimulation using magnets.

What we all need to remember as we look ahead to medicine in this new century is that there has been a big shift from acute to chronic illnesses and that degenerative conditions, including cancer, heart disease and diabetes, are all on the increase in the West. And these are exactly the kinds of conditions that complementary medicine can work with, alongside orthodox practice.

We should not turn our back on 100 years' worth of progress in medical science, but neither should we dismiss treatments for which clinical evidence is still scanty simply on the basis that we do not believe what we cannot touch or see.

Quantum physics has already taught us this lesson: when you look at a stone you see a cold, inert mass, but scrutinise that same stone under a microscope and you'll see a mass of frantic activity as electrons vibrate and fly around. Even more extraordinary, physics has shown that the very act of looking at something changes its fundamental nature.

Inert or moving? It's your world. You decide.

Animal Magic

Connecting Back to Nature and a Sacred Life

My life changed in a curious way, but definitely for the better, the day I found a baby blackbird in the lane alongside the beech woods opposite my house. It had clearly fallen out of the nest, but there were no protective parents around. After a long internal debate, I decided to bring it home with me. The bird lived on my porch for several weeks until it was strong enough to fly away. Aside from the pleasure of feeding it, it taught me one of life's most valuble lessons: Trust and have faith in life as it unfolds.

Did you know that every single day of its life the blackbird sings before dawn?

Think about it. This unobtrusive backyard bird, which so many of us ignore and take for granted when we see it swooping across our lawns, knows something that so many people spend their whole life missing. Like all those animals who live alongside us, either in the wild or as our domesticated pets, birds have an innate wisdom about their place in the grand scheme of things and about how life will follow the grand plan.

I have been lucky enough to have met, in person, some of the world's most respected spiritual teachers and health gurus. One person who helped set me on a journey of discovery about the richness of the shamanic healing traditions, including the crucial role of animal totems even in everyday, modern lives, was the writer, broadcaster and now shamanic practitioner Leslie Kenton, whose very name is synonymous with glowing good health and well-being.

Having attended several shamanic workshops, I do not subscribe to the currently fashionable theory that each and every one of us is a latent shamanic healer, if we did but know it, but I do believe, without question, that we can all benefit from this ancient wisdom in our 21st-century lives. Shamans or medicine men and -women believe that all illness and disease is a manifestation of a spiritual demise. They seek, then, to heal the spirit of a person as well as and even before treating the physical symptoms.

There has been an explosion of interest in the subject over the last few years – and when you realise that shamanic traditions have their roots all over the world, in Europe among the ancient Celts and in Africa and Asia, and not just in South America, you can understand how it is that some of this ancient knowledge remains in our very bloodlines.

Leslie Kenton, who has studied all the world's major religions and healing techniques in a lifetime devoted to whole health, says she has chosen the shamanic route herself because you get results, fast. The 'result' she and other practitioners talk about refer to the information they glean when they embark on what is known as a shamanic journey. This is a 'journey' into the spiritual realms, which may seem unreal to many but which is, to the shaman, as real as any experience in this reality which we call daily life (and they call the middle world).

They may travel, for example, to the lower world (or underworld) , a place inhabited by spirit guides, often in the form of what is called a power animal, who will then journey with them, helping them seek out the information and guidance they need. They may choose to travel to the more ethereal upper world, what we might call heaven, to talk to more angelic and heavenly creatures of wisdom and light. What they will always do is travel with a specific question in mind and the altruistic purpose of bringing back information for the greater good (of the tribe, in indigenous cultures, or for a particular individual who is in need). What they must never do is journey with the wrong motives, including their own selfish gain or with the aim of causing harm to another.

Before you dismiss the idea of other realities as a load of gibberish, ask yourself how you can explain the fact that all those who journey regularly report back an almost identical landscape? The obvious answer is they must have seen a map in a book somewhere. How, then, do we explain the fact that cultures as diverse as the ancient Celts and the Native American tribes all practised shamanism too and used the same altered-state-of-consciousness techniques to learn more about true healing?

How To Journey

Many indigenous cultures use psychotropic plants to induce the state of altered consciousness that is a pre-requisite for a shamanic journey. One of the favoured plants is Ayahuasca which will change your brain chemistry to bring about this altered mental state. In the West, we tend to use drumming to change the patterns of the brainwaves and achieve the same altered state. Research has shown how the brainwaves alter in deep meditation (see Chapter 10) and scientific studies now show rhythmic drumming does the same thing, only faster.

If you are alone, you will need a drumming tape. If you are in a drumming group, elect one person to drum and everyone else should prepare to journey. First, decide whether you are going to visit the upper or the lower world. Most beginners find it easier to start with the latter. There is nothing negative or sinister about this world, so do not be alarmed. You will not come to any harm. Decide on a place that is known to you in this reality, to act as a portal down into the earth. It could be, for example, a cave you have visited, a deep well outside your home, a staircase down to a cellar or even the exposed roots of an ancient tree in the woods that you will trace, in your mind, deep into the ground.

This must be a real place, not somewhere in your imagination. It will also be the route via which you always enter and leave the lower world. Now make sure you are going to be comfortable. Spread a blanket on the ground and tie a scarf or a piece of fabric over your eyes to block out any daylight or other distractions. If you don't have a scarf, simply cover your eyes with your arm. Lie down and take yourself, in your mind, to the place that is your entrance to the lower world.

As you get used to the drumbeat, begin your descent, knowing you are completely safe. You may meet creatures along the way who want to help you. That's fine. Thank them for their concern and continue along your way. The purpose of this first journey is to get an idea of the landscape and then come straight back. After 15 or 20 minutes, whatever you have agreed beforehand, you will hear what is called the Call Back. This is signalled by a change in the rhythm of the drumming that you have all agreed beforehand. Do not ignore this but stop and retrace your steps back to the place where you entered.

Lots of people report the sensation of spiralling down a tunnel when they do this exercise for the first time. Others say nothing happened and they didn't see anything. I even know a woman who reported that she had to go back to bed, in her mind, to get started and who conducted her first journey peering out from the duvet cover. There is no right or wrong. As with everything in life, you will find the experience improves with practice.

One of the most important tools in developing the link with this ancient knowledge and in starting to incorporate it into your everyday life is the 'bridge' between this reality and the worlds you visit while undertaking a shamanic journey. To build this bridge, when you return remain silent for 5 or 10 minutes, however long you need to record through words, drawings or a simple diary your impressions and the details of your journey.

How It Worked for Me

There is, as always, no substitute for experience. You can read every book on shamanism in the land and still not really understand its potency. I had two experiences that convinced me it really works. I was, as I mentioned earlier, attending one of Leslie Kenton's popular shamanic workshops in London. It was the last day of the two-day course and Leslie asked us to work in pairs to go on a shamanic journey and return with a power animal for our partner.

Since I had absolutely no confidence I could do anything of the sort, I asked for a partner who already had a power animal and so would not be disappointed if I failed in the mission. In other words, I wanted someone who was already experienced in shamanic techniques. We completed this exercise and my partner brought me back a giraffe. This, she said, symbolised taking a long-distance outlook on life. With its long neck and high head, the giraffe, she explained, can see what lies ahead, is very sociable and has a third horn located just above the eyes, in the same place as the mystical third eye.

I liked what she said but was not at all convinced. Leslie then told us, as we left, that our power animal would make itself known and make its presence felt. I travelled home that night on the London underground and, while waiting for a train, looked up to see an enormous advertising hoarding in a colour I could only described as giraffe-yellow. I decided I was tired and needed to get a grip on myself, especially when I reached the mainline station only to see half of it sectioned off for building works with partition boards in the exactly same colour. Two days later, my sister Melissa called me to say my then 3-year-old niece, Tiana, had done a drawing for me and was insisting she post it to me. This had never happened before, so I asked what she had drawn. You've guessed it. Her yellow giraffe is in my office where I write, and I have a beautifully carved wooden one in the house which always reminds me to take the long-distance look of life, to avoid the short-term knee-jerk reaction and to see the whole picture, not just what is under my nose.

During another shamanic journey, I came across a feathery plant which told me it was Yarrow. At that time I could not have pointed out a yarrow plant in the hedgerow despite it being a native of both England and America, and I could not have drawn you the shape of its leaves. I asked the plant what it was for, and was surprised when it answered me back in an East End Cockney accent, 'For what you got now.' I had, at the time, severe menstrual cramps and was in some discomfort. At the end of the journey I drew an image of what I had seen in my bridge-building journal, and made a note to check the description in a herbal. You already know what I am going to tell you. The leaves are, as I had drawn, feathery, and if you read up on the plant you'll find it has an ancient use in staunching bloodflow, especially menstruation and cramping.

Some people will dismiss this as simply an over-vivid imagination, of course. I say, so what if it is? You are still accessing the source of something both powerful and mystical, and once you become experienced, something potentially useful to yourself and others. After a great deal of subsequent research into the subject, my experience with yarrow was, I now believe, me simply tapping into an ancient knowledge that is carried in all our genetic material (DNA and RNA). You carry that same ancient knowledge yourself, and can learn to do the same thing. What I do not propound is the idea that we can all become shamanic healers, which I believe, with the odd exception to the rule, requires dedication and rigorous training over a lifetime in the skills and techniques of this ancient practice.

The first time I journeyed, nothing happened and I almost gave up. Typically, I was told, high achievers and those who over-intellectualise will have problems at the outset. But on the third or fourth occasion, I had the experience I have reported here which, if nothing else, taught me to take Yarrow tincture when I have menstrual cramps.

Animals as Totems

The shamans believe that each of us is born with nine animals who bring us teachings and messages to help us live our lives with a greater understanding of our own journey. Two of these animals are permanent and will never leave us. They are our primary totem, otherwise known as our Power Animals.

We usually know instinctively which animals they are. We will feel drawn to them throughout our lives and may often dream of them. One walks on the left to guard and guide our feminine energies; the other walks on the right to protect our masculine characteristics.

It is important to remember that these animals choose you, not the other way around. Lots of people think they can choose an animal and start linking with it, but it does not work that way. No animal is better or worse than any other. Each animal has its own unique medicine, and you will get your best results by accepting with thanks the one that comes to you.

If you think you already know your animal totems, check through the following questions.

> **Which animal or bird has always fascinated you?**
> **When you visited the zoo as a child, which animal did you want to visit most and first?**
> **What animals do you see most of in nature? Have you encountered any in the wild?**
> **Of all the animals in the world, which one interests you right now?**

Which animal frightens you most?

Have you ever been bitten or attacked by an animal? (The shamans believe if you survive an attack, this is your spirit animal.)

Which animals appear in your dreams (especially recurring ones)?

Finding Your Own Power Animal

To find your own power animal, you will need to journey to the lower world with the sole intention of meeting him or her. This will be your only task. Prepare to journey as described above. You may meet many animals and creatures along the way, but your personal power animal will make more than one appearance. As a general guideline, if the same animal crops up four times, this is the one you will be bringing home with you.

When I say it will make an appearance, do not expect the kind of image you might see in a David Attenborough film. The spirit realms have a highly developed sense of humour, and spiritual gifts are not given without you doing a little work to merit them. If your power animal is a rabbit, for example, you may just catch a glimpse of a bobtail behind a rock. You might then see what looks like a cartoon image of Roger Rabbit out of the corner of your eye. Your rabbit totem may then turn up as the Easter Bunny or you might see its image as a sculpture or a work of art.

You may start your journey hoping to come back with a glamorous, soaring eagle, a wise old owl or an intelligent dolphin, but don't be surprised if you get a mouse, a mongoose or even a mandarin duck. Whatever you get will be the right power animal for you at this time in your life. Eventually, you will discover you have several power animals and these can come and go in your life, just like human friends. The only creatures you must not bring back are snakes showing their fangs, fish with spikes, or spiders. Otherwise, anything goes.

Taking Clues from Your New Guide

In his fantastic book *Animal-Speak*, the author and shaman Ted Andrews explains how you can read the symbolism of not just which power animal has assigned itself to you, but of all the animals you come across in your life. Just as my baby blackbird taught me the meaning of faith, so a creature that passes your way can tell you something about your life. You can interpret the meaning of its colour and even, once you become skilled in reading animal signs, the importance of the direction from which it appeared.

You may also want to study this creature's own native habitat to learn more about its significance in your life. Even its feeding and mating habits may give you some clues. Your power animal will also probably start to show up in your daily life, just as my giraffe did. You may catch sight of it on an item of TV news or in a book someone else has borrowed from the library. The important thing to remember is that this animal is on your side. The shamanic theory is that the power animals are spirits who have lived in this reality we call the real world and who know how hard it can be to cut it here. They want to help and have probably been waiting to make your acquaintance. They often have an excellent sense of humour and are playful and, according to tradition, will love it if you make a special place for them in your life by putting a picture of them on your wall or fridge or by thinking about them when you meditate or are simply relaxing in the bath.

What Different Animals Mean

So, once you've mastered the art of shamanic journeying and found the power animal that in shamanic tradition is said to have been waiting for you all along, how do you figure out what it might mean?

Your own intuition will tell you a great deal about the significance of your animal totem. If, for example, you have a raven, you may need to think about developing your own psychic abilities. Linked by many cultures with the mystery of death, the raven is associated with clairvoyance. If you have a mouse, the message may be that you are so busy concentrating on the big things in life, you are not paying attention to the all-important small details. You may be diluting your energies by scattering them and trying to do too much at the same time.

The following table is really only a signpost for some of the animal totems. To really understand yours, find out everything you can about how that animal lives, what it eats, where it sleeps, how it survives and plays. Its significance in your life will soon become clear.

Animal	Significance
Alligator	Man is the alligator's only enemy. It has enormous powers to survive and digs deep burrows when the waters are high, so that it has a wet nest in the dry season. Maybe you need to plan ahead more.

Badger	Badgers live in simple but very clean dens and bring the gift of tidiness and good organisation. Badger medicine is bold but gets results. These magical creatures never surrender and teach the importance of self-reliance and trust.
Butterfly	Butterflies may look fragile, but some can migrate up to 3000 miles. Whenever an ecosystem is damaged or destroyed, they are the first creatures to leave. They signify balance and teach that change does not have to be traumatic.
Deer	One of my favourites, the deer teaches strength through gentleness and the importance of unconditional love. A stag with antlers may be a sign to tune in to your higher self to find your soul's true purpose.
Dolphin	Living their lives in a harmonious community, dolphins, with their huge brains have much to teach man. A symbol of salvation to the early Christians, the dolphin encourages us to play and to find more balance in our lives.
Eagle	The sacred messenger, shamanic healers often work with eagle feathers. The Golden Eagle flies higher than any other bird. One of the most admired birds and a symbol of great power, its message is all about spiritual healing.

Elephant	The largest living land mammal, the elephant is a symbol of royalty and fertility. Their trunks confer an exceptional sense of smell to help them discriminate good from bad. If an elephant is your totem, you may want to re-establish a strong sense of family and community.
Fox	To get rid of fleas, a fox will take a stick into its mouth and submerge itself slowly in water, which fleas hate. As the fox sinks, the fleas leap off its coat to the nearest dry thing – the stick in its mouth. Pure genius. If a fox, with all its beauty and charm, has shown up in your life it may be telling you to adopt a lower profile and be more discreet.
Horse	No other animal has played a greater role in the civilization of man. The horse is the symbol of freedom and spiritual life. Is it time to move on in your life?
Lion	The second-largest of the big cats, the lion is a symbol of the sun. The female is the better hunter. If this is your animal, trust your more female side – creativity and intuition.
Magpie	Probably the most intelligent of the crows, the magpie reminds of us of the duality of life. If I give you a beautiful ring, I also give give you the fear of losing it. Linked with earth magic and the craft of the wise, this

bird is independent-minded and has a strong will of its own.

Owl

The Hopi tribe believe owls are the teachers of the medicine of the night. In ancient Celtic shamanism, the owl signifies seeing through the darkness to the spiritual light. Owl people can often see the darkness in other people's souls which is not a gift everyone would welcome. If you have the owl, then keeping quiet and getting on with your life will bring its own rewards.

Rabbit

I once hand-raised a baby rabbit that had been injured by a passing car. I hated to let him go but once he was mobile again, he hopped off through the bluebell woods. I admired his courage since the rabbit faces so many everyday dangers. It is also one of the most fertile creatures on the planet and has much to teach about survival. They are skilled at keeping out of sight and can keep themselves perfectly still if they have to.

Rat

It beats me why people still hate and fear rats so much. Intelligent and able to reason, the wild rats are even brighter than the poor laboratory ones. Those born under the Chinese astrological sign of the rat are said to be heading for success. A rat in your life may also warn you are working too hard.

Squirrel

Squirrels learn by copying and as a totem, tell you it may be better to learn by doing than reading about something. Sociable and bursting with an excitable energy, they have much to teach about getting ready for each phase of your life.

Wolf

A powerful totem that speaks of the importance of ritual and loyalty. These wonderful creatures live by rules and hierarchy in their community. Wolf experts have reported a special relationship between ravens and wolves. If the wolf is your totem, tune in to your own spiritual wisdom and inner life.

Meditation & Prayer

If the only prayer you say in your whole life is 'thank you'
that would be enough.

Meister Eckhart

Meditation – Why Bother?

The first time somebody suggested I make time to meditate, I thought the woman was stark raving mad – especially when she suggested I set aside an hour a day. 'I DON'T HAVE TIME FOR THAT' I yelled, just to make sure she understood just how very busy I was. And that, she said quietly, was exactly her point.

It would have been tempting to dismiss this woman as an old hippy, but there was no whiff of patchouli oil or a single love bead in sight. Instead, she was power-dressed in an expensive designer suit, sporting a sleek blonde bob and promoting her new book, which was all about bringing balance back into over-busy lives.

I had found the book inspiring, and so decided to give this meditation thing I kept hearing people rave about a try. Imagine my disappointment when I found that having plonked onto the cold floor in a painful cross-legged position, I could not do it. I tried closing my eyes, chanting *om* and emptying my mind, but it just didn't work.

First, an almighty 'to do' list rushed to mind. Then I remembered I had forgotten to buy dog food. My mind wandered to an imaginary confrontation with the bank manager, and quickly drifted from that unsavoury topic to wonder whatever happened to my first love. After 5 minutes, by which time my hips were killing me, I gave up.

This would be funny if it was not utterly typical of the experience of most Westerners trying to meditate for the first time. You do, I realised, discover something very extraordinary about life during that very first attempt, but far from floating into a dreamlike state where the deepest secrets of the universe are revealed to you, you find that sitting perfectly still is about the most agonising thing you are ever likely to try. Worse, even if you ignore the pain, emptying your mind is simply beyond the scope and imagination of most of us.

What helped to turn my own meditation practice around was the good fortune of meeting a teacher who showed me how to concentrate on the rise and fall of the breath alone. She told me how she disliked the idea of meditation as a solely spiritual practice and saw it, instead, as a life tool that is available to everyone who wants to strengthen their inner life and make what she calls more mindful choices.

The Benefits

The words meditate, medicine and medicate all share the same Latin root – *medicus* – meaning 'to cure' and anyone who has made meditation part of their everyday life will be able to bore for their country with the long, long list of all its proven health benefits.

As far back as the early 1970s, scientists were able to monitor how meditation changes the pattern of brainwaves from the busy, everyday beta-waves to the slower alpha-waves, thus inducing a calmer, more reflective and healthier state of mind and muscle tone.

Other health benefits, now all well documented too, include lowering cholesterol levels, reducing high blood pressure and all its associated risks, banishing stress, relieving depression, increasing self-confidence and even helping to reverse arteriosclerosis, the medical term for arteries that have hardened as a result of plaque deposits, usually due to poor lifestyle choices.

In other words, meditation bestows almost perfect health.

You do not need special clothes to meditate, or even a special chair (although Monk-style meditation stools are popular). You can do it anytime, anywhere and it won't leave you feeling puffed and out of breath. It is the perfect antidote to the non-stop demands of 21st-century life, so why don't more of us incorporate daily meditation into our lives?

One reason is that our logical brain finds it hard to accept just sitting still can bring any benefits at all. In modern life we want our miracle cures and we want them now. We do not want to have to work at them or practise anything to get good at it. This is why, of the thousands of Westeners who take up some form of meditation every week, most have given up within the first year, which is a shame since the more you practise meditation, the greater the benefits.

How to Sit Still for More than Five Minutes without Screaming

My own practice got back on track when I learned a meditation technique called *Vipassana*, which means 'insight'. That said, it does not really matter what technique you practise. I personally like this one because of its simplicity.

Said to have been taught and practised by Buddha himself, *Vipassana* is not a theology but a means to an end. And it could not be more simple. You do not chant *om* or any other mantra. You do not focus your gaze on a candle flame until your eyes water, nor do you have to find your mystical Third Eye. You simply allow yourself to sit still, back straight, eyes shut, and to shut out the external world by following the rise and fall of your own breathing.

You are also, thankfully, allowed to pad your bottom with cushions which will tilt the pelvis forward so your knees come closer to the ground, allowing your hips to open gently and remain more comfortable in the cross-legged position. You can even move, if you think the pain of keeping still will kill you, although the reason you are encouraged to sit through such discomfort is that it teaches you the value of impermanence. Nothing in the world stays the same; that maddening itch behind your ear or the excruciating pain in your hip will pass. Meditation helps you learn to notice such discomforts, but not to become attached to them.

To derive all the full benefits of meditation, you need to build up to sitting for at least 20 minutes at a time. Your legs may feel numb and you may have to suffer pins and needles when you do move at the end of it, but the feeling of being centred and connected again will be more than worth it.

What remains difficult for most beginners, is the idea of complete stillness. Doing nothing has been all but eradicated from our daily lives. We spend so much time on automatic pilot or concentrating on one aspect of our day, usually to the detriment of everything else, that we rarely take time to notice and absorb our surroundings. We are so used to the constant stimulation of all our senses that, if this were to stop, we would probably question whether we were still alive.

The reason for this stillness is to allow you to reconnect with your own inner life and your true self. Most of us do not see ourselves through our own eyes. We are someone else's wife, brother, mother, sister, work colleague, team mate or boss. This detachment from our own inner world robs of us our connection with our true self – the self that knows what is best for us, how to achieve it and what to do once we have.

A lot of people who are new to meditation complain, just as I first did, that it just does not work for them. I am not sure exactly what I was expecting, but I know now that to say 'I cannot do it' is missing the entire point. If meditation is about anything at all, it is the idea of *being* and not doing.

There is no right or wrong, because whatever comes up for you is exactly what needs to come up. If nothing happens, accept it. If you feel a momentary insight into the wonderfulness of life and your connection to all things, be thankful for it.

Chants and Mantras

Most people take up some form of chanting through yoga or meditation – although if you stop to think about it, many Westerners get their first introduction to chanting in childhood when attending church.

Once you are comfortable with the practice of meditation, the aim is to then use a mantra to help to still the mind further from its incessant chatter. This will not only bring you peace, poise and inner strength but will even bring you closer to God since, according to the mystics, God can only speak to you and you can only hear Him when your mind is still and empty. Study any of the spiritual scriptures and they all reach this same conclusion, no matter what form of God it is they worship. If you want to connect to the divine, you need to make room for some silence in your life.

The most powerful of all the one-word mantras is the word *Aum*. These three sounds, *a*, *u* and *m*, are said to represent the three states of waking, dreaming and sleeping respectively. And according to NASA scientists, they represent something else – the recorded sound of the whole universe, which has now been captured on tape.

It is the vibrational energy of the mantra you chant, not the word itself, that is said to cleanse all negative energy and connect you back to your own God. The more times a mantra is chanted, the stronger its spiritual energy. The idea is that if you chant or simply repeat your chosen mantra in silence to yourself, you can bring your mind to a level of inner awareness which will transform both your inner and outer life.

The word *mantra* comes from the root *man*, meaning 'to think', and *trai*, meaning 'to protect [or free] from the bondage of this world'. One interpretation is that a mantra is a thought that both liberates and protects you. Lots of people choose Sanskrit mantras because Sanskrit is a sacred language, but you can choose any word or phrase that is sacred to and has a special meaning for you.

Devotees of chanting claim that its physical benefits include lowering blood pressure and improved cardiovascular health. It can also, if you persevere for some time, help you reach an altered state of consciousness. Since chanting prolongs the exhalation of the breath, it also calms the mind. You can feel its power when you chant in a room full of likeminded people, say in a yoga class, and it can also give you a true sense of how you are in yourself. It is deeply purifying and I often find I feel nauseated after a Chanting class.

In yoga we learn that each chakra (or energy centre) contains a 'seed' (or *biji*) sound that can also be used as a mantra. Chant one of these and you will feel or sense the sound of the vibration activating the energy of that chakra.

The sound for the root or base chakra, for instance, is *Lam*. The sound for the lower abdomen chakra is *Vam*. To energise the solar plexus chakra behind the naval, chant *Ram*, and to vibrate with the heart chakra, chant *Yam*. The chakra of communication lies in the throat and is activated when you chant *Ham*. The brow chakra (or mystical Third Eye) is energised by the mantra *Om*, which also activates the crown chakra. (For chakra healing, see page 277.)

The Nepalese Good Luck Mantra

This mantra was sent anonymously to me. If you are looking for instructions for life, you will find these hard to beat.

1. **Remember that great love and great achievements involve great risk.**
2. **When you lose, don't lose the lesson.**
3. **Follow the three Rs:**
    - **respect for yourself**
    - **respect for others**
    - **responsibility for all your actions.**
4. **Realise that not getting what you want is sometimes a wonderful stroke of luck.**
5. **Learn the rules so you know how to break them properly.**

6. Don't let a little dispute injure a great friendship.

7. When you realise you have made a mistake, take immediate steps to correct it.

8. Spend some time alone every day.

9. Open your arms to change, but don't let go of your values.

10. Remember that silence is sometimes the best answer.

11. Live a good and honourable life. Then, when you get older and think back, you'll be able to enjoy it all over again.

12. A loving atmosphere in your home is the foundation for your life.

13. In disagreements with loved ones, deal only with the current situation. Don't bring up the past.

14. Share your knowledge. It's the way to achieve immortality.

15. Be gentle with the earth.

16. Once a year, go somewhere you have not been before.

17. Remember that the best relationship is one where your love for each other exceeds your need for each other.

18. Judge your success by what you have to give up to get it.

19. Approach love and cooking with the same reckless abandon.

20. Pass this on to those you love. It is the energy we give something, by thought and belief, that empowers it.

Prayer, Peace & Quiet

Prayer Feeds The Soul —
as blood is to the body,
prayer is to the soul —
and it brings you closer to God

Mother Teresa, Everything Starts from Prayer

It is not just your soul that likes prayer. The body seems to respond just as positively, according to researchers. Psychologists, reporting in the *British Journal of Health Psychology*, found that personal prayer, more than going to church or being religious, was an excellent way of promoting well-being.

These researchers questioned almost 500 UK students about their religious leanings, the frequency of personal prayer in their lives, and church attendance. They also measured depressive symptoms, anxiety and self-esteem.
What they found was that those individuals who prayed daily or more often were more likely to report lower rates of depression, lower levels of anxiety and higher self-esteem than those who only ever prayed when things went wrong in their lives.

A prayer is just a silent conversation with whatever divine power you recognise. Call it God or the higher self, it doesn't really matter. What does count is the proven impact of prayer, which, far from being an old-fashioned superstition and an insurance blanket against the faint possibility that there might just turn out to be something more to life, can dramatically affect not only your own well-being but all those around you.

In his introduction to Mother Teresa's book, *Everything Starts From Prayer*, Larry Dossey, the American physician and himself the author of *Healing Words*, *Prayer Is Good Medicine*, reports that the physical body itself likes prayer so much so that scientific studies have shown, again and again, that both the cardiovascular and the immune systems appear to be strengthened by it. Of course, he stresses, for a prayer to work it must be done with good intentions and unconditional love.

The Spiritual Journey

As we celebrate the first years of a new millennium, there has been a massive shift in consciousness in the West. A growing number of non-religious people are beginning to see and treat their lives as, above all else, a spiritual journey. These people hold down ordinary jobs and probably don't even go to church or the mosque regularly, but they know there is something more to life and can't resist the call to find it.

It is for people like this that a worldwide scheme called National Quiet Day was first introduced in 1994, and that a charity called The Quiet Garden Trust, which is also promoted by The National Retreat Association, was launched. The Quiet Garden Trust aims to introduce people to their own spiritual path through the beauty of nature, and now has 166 'spaces' worldwide where you can just sit and *be*.

The whole of creation, whether it's the thunder of the sea below a cliff, the sight of a bluebell wood in April or the unfurling of new leaves on a young tree in the spring, seems to strike a deep chord with people. The purpose of the Quiet Garden Trust is to provide somewhere for people to go and be reflective.

Connecting back with nature is both reassuring and spiritually rejuvenating. We begin to recognise how nature carries on with her cycles regardless of what we do or what is happening to us. It is this sense of perspective that is often helpful to people as they struggle to make this inner journey in their lives. Making time for spiritual reflection in a garden can help root and ground people in a very literal way – and for city dwellers who usually see nothing but concrete, the Garden Trust can provide access to something that is beautiful and growing.

For some, though, the idea of a silent retreat is too daunting, even if it only lasts a day. If enforced silence makes you nervous, try a Guided Quiet Day. This means, instead of arriving and plunging straight into the strange atmosphere of silence between strangers, there is an experienced speaker who will discuss some aspect of spiritual life and allow short periods of time for silent reflection on his or her comments.

The subject on the first-ever Quiet Day I attended was 'symbols of pilgrimage'. If you look upon life as a spiritual journey, then this was a talk which could have been given just as easily at a New Age Mind/Body/Spirit festival or in church. The speaker, American-born Jo Durrell, spoke of the dove as a symbol of purity, fire as a sign of cleansing, wind as the breath of life and light as the symbol of truth and the vision ahead. The emphasis was on Christian prayer, but you are at liberty to follow your own path and if you want to meditate or even fall asleep, that's fine.

I certainly felt this was an excellent introduction to the idea of being quiet in a safe place with no pressure to perform. I felt there were fewer expectations of me than if I'd been stepping into a church, and I knew I was in no way stuck there (which is a risk when you go to a retreat in the middle of nowhere). There was no mad banging of tambourines or zealous chanting, and I felt perfectly welcome, comfortable and, most importantly, still – the very thing I had been seeking – throughout.

If you still prefer the idea of being quiet on your own, then you might like to investigate one of the new Centres for Reflection springing up to cater for those seeking greater spiritual connection. In the UK, the number of these has already reached double figures. Attending one, you'd be forgiven for thinking you're actually in a church-by-any-other-name, because you will be since the number of churches now opening their doors as such centres is growing.

Going On Retreat

Retreat leaders often shake their heads when they see a new 'retreatant' sauntering up the path dragging a massive holdall full of books, magazines and CDs, because the whole idea of a Quiet Day or retreat is to shed the clutter that fills your everyday life and make space for new realisations which can help you on your spiritual journey through life.

What I discovered in my own quest for some serious peace and quiet was that the retreat movement has changed. Many of the big retreat houses, especially those run by religious orders whose members have grown elderly, have closed due to a lack of physical and financial resources. In their place, the idea of the small house retreat has blossomed. Here, ordinary people open some part of their home or a converted outbuilding or barn to just two or three retreatants at a time. There will be no organised events as such, but there is always someone available to discuss your reflections with you and, perhaps, suggest books which could help you on your path.

The Path You Take

Examine the underlying principle of any of the world's great religions and you will find what the writer Aldous Huxley called *the Perennial Philosophy*, which appears in every age and every civilisation. First, there is an infinite and changeless reality beneath the world of change. Secondly, this same reality lies at the core of every human personality. Thirdly, the purpose of life is to discover this reality, experientially, for yourself and thus to realise God in whatever form you believe while you are here on earth.

The early Christian mystics knew this. So did the Indian sages. Mother Teresa devoted her life to sharing this knowledge. Gandhi knew it was the only path to peace, as did St Paul, who said: 'Someone who is joined to the Lord is one spirit.'

It is not a philosophy of the East or the West, but of the whole spiritual world. Everyone who comes to know this has done so through the only possible route – silence. The Christians call it comtemplation. To the Buddhists it is meditation. One of the greatest revelations in my life was realising, through my yoga practice and study, that they are all talking about the exact same thing.

The point about life is that you are not seperate from a vengeful God who will not listen to or answer your prayers. Instead, when you take time out to listen, you realise your God is not only real and compassionate but everywhere. With this realisation comes the knowledge that the world is not made up of pieces but is a whole that is a manifestation of God. Once you know this, you know too that while your physical body will one day die, the inner you will go on forever.

I like the way the *Bhagavad Gita*, a cornerstone of the Hindu religion and the yogic philosophy, describes this: 'Once you have realised the essential immortality that is the birthright of every human being, then death is no more traumatic than taking off an old coat.'

What I like even more is the fact that science, in the form of quantum physics, has proved what the mystics knew all along – that we are all connected, all part of the Divine, and that we can learn to create our own lives.

Time Out

'Time out' is a much-used phrase. We all know what it means, but few of us take it seriously enough to make space for it in our lives. This is a shame, since you can only make true changes and real progress in your inner life when you step off the mad whirlygig of your everyday life long enough to figure out where you want to go, how you're going to get there, and why it's important to chill out along the way.

I am not actually, as it turns out, a huge fan of organised and traditional spa breaks. Aside from the fact that I, personally, find more peace from solitude and being connected to the natural world, many spas, especially the so-called health farms, need dragging firmly into the 21st century. I have had the misfortune to be in places where microwaved stodgy canelloni swimming in a milk-based cheese sauce is considered a wholesome lunch, and where grated salad and coleslaw is offered up as the salad option. I have literally had to run from novice therapists who would have happily slapped any old mix of oils on my face, and I have been appalled by limp-wristed, delicate-looking women who have decided healing is their true vocation and who affect to be able to offer up any of the benefits of a good massage, Ayurvedic or Western.

That said, if you know the right places to go, the ones to avoid and what to expect when you get there, a spa break can work wonders for your physical and spiritual well-being.

Where to Go?

Before deciding where to go to take Time Out, do your homework. You cannot beat a good word-of-mouth recommendation, and if a friend has had a fantastic time at a spa or retreat ask as many questions as you can to see if it would suit you too.

If you have never done any yoga or meditation, then a 10-day astanga workshop on a yacht sailing around the Caribbean may sound thrilling but may be something of a baptism of fire, especially if you are not physically fit. You may love the sound of a spa that is on the other side of the world, but there is no point rushing over there on a long weekend break, trying to squeeze in every activity that is on offer and coming home feeling frazzled, jet-lagged and as if something is still missing. This is not the point of any spa or retreat break.

If you are going to join a guided-workshop-type break, check out the teacher first. Some of the world's top spiritual gurus do lead small groups to sacred places around the globe, but remember you are going to be stuck with these people for up to two weeks. Some of them will not only be demanding centre-stage, but will also be pretty intent on reliving earlier traumas in their lives so that they can come home feeling reborn. This might be great for them, but it could prove a little tiresome for you.

Some people feel worried about the idea of a silent retreat. Again, if this makes you feel uncomfortable, don't plunge straight in. I have been on retreats where we have had all our meals in silence, and I have to say that sitting at a table with complete strangers and not being able to rely on the usual conversational gambits or social etiquette to make yourself feel more comfortable is tough. The first time I experienced the initial embarrassment of this, I couldn't wait to nod my excuses and leave – but it begins to feel more comfortable the more you do it.

The What Really Works Top Time Out Breaks

As the Mind & Body launch editor of the Freespirited.com Internet travel site, I have sifted through hundreds of spa reviews in my search for those places that really know how to help their visitors nurture their inner life, as well as their physical body.

We have a talented team of top health writers who have travelled the globe to find the best spiritual and spa retreats for weary bodies and souls. Eventually, though, finding the place that appeals to you most is a very personal choice.

You might like the sound of a spa that is on your own doorstep, or you might prefer to travel halfway across the world to mingle with the jet set and spend five days being massaged by highly skilled therapists who have spent seven years training with monks in the Buddhist monasteries of Thailand. This may sound irresistably glamorous when you are flicking through the glossy travel brochure from the comfort of your own home, but remember there will be no exciting nightlife or shopping; if you are used to more diversions, the shock of being stuck for a week in a remote hill station retreat might leave you feeling disorientated, homesick and downright bored, however good the masseurs.

There are spas to suit every budget, and plenty of guide books with all the details you could ever want and more. What I have done here and in keeping with my investigations for *What Really Works* is to make a very personal selection of some of the more secret places you can slip away to as part of your rejuvenation of a tired body and soul. Most I have been to myself, and cannot wait to revisit. Others are on my wish-list, the kind of places that my mind drifts off to when the deadlines come crowding in and when any kind of break seems a very remote possibility. It may not seem so on the surface, but each of them has something very special and unique to offer the tired, world-weary or those simply seeking to rest the body and soul.

This is not guide book hyperbole. None of these places knows that they are being included on this list. Many will not even fit most people's idea of a spa or retreat, but don't let that put you off. The beautifying mud treatments at The

Institute of Yoga in Lonavala, India, for example, use a cow dung paste – but you don't come here for the pampering, rather perhaps to experience yoga in its homeland and definitely to meet the Institute's inspirational spiritual leader, who is known as *Swamiji*.

Galleon Beach in Antigua looks for all the world like any other palm-fringed holiday resort, but it would be hard to beat the quiet practice of yoga on the balcony as the sun rises and the sea laps its way almost to the front door of your airy and unpretentious cottage.

For an introduction to true shamanism and its powerful healing traditions, the little-known Wilka t'ika in Peru will call to your soul from somewhere very deep. If you've been stuck in London all week and can't wait to escape to rediscover just what your spiritual life is all about, you will love St Katherine's at Parmoor in Oxfordshire. Take time to sit among the graves of the priests and nuns who have been associated with this place and feel the call of your own spiritual beliefs.

For contact details, see Resources.

The Institute of Yoga, Lonavala, India

This hospital, yoga college and retreat centre is three hours by bus from Bombay. The grounds may be lush but the Institute is next to a very busy road. The noise never stops, day or night, but this is India for the true spiritual traveller. The ashram is a collection of slightly shabby single-, two- and three-storey buildings. The accommodation is basic but clean. The Ayurvedic food is simple but nutritious, and if you're here for spiritual rejuvenation you will not leave disappointed. Swamiji is an unassuming, wise and profoundly holy man, who gives freely of his time and wisdom. His stories will remind you exactly of why you are here. His message to Westerners is a very clear one: Don't walk away from your own world to spread the word, but practise your spiritual beliefs through example in your own daily life. Don't miss the twice-daily Fire Ceremony prayer rituals or this yogic Swami who both understands the pressures of 21st-century Western living and who, refreshingly for a guru, laughs at his own jokes!

Shamrock Cottage, Galleon Beach, Antigua

Here, you can rent your own small corner of paradise to meditate, practise yoga or warm your body in a sun that will help you store up vitamin D supplies for winter. These are the only self-catering cottages actually on the beachfront on the whole of this cricket-mad island, and this is the one with a palm tree right outside your bedroom window. Because you're self-catering, you can chill out with a sea and sand break and still ensure your diet stays healthy. One tip, though, the supermarkets are not stocked with as many of the beans, grains or pulses that you might need, so take the precaution of packing some of your own healthfoods before you leave home. What the stores lack in convenience foods, the island more than makes up for with exotic fruits, so start your day with a generous fruit bowl. Forget the glamour of the reputation of this Caribbean idyll. So what if Eric Clapton has a hilltop home here? He also has a drug rehabilitation centre, and for as much offshore money as there is swilling around there is also a lot of poverty. The infrastructure and poor state of the roads makes hiring a jeep the most sensible option. If you stay here on the beach, you can organise your car hire through Ti Ti, who owns and runs Colombo's, the Italian restaurant behind the cottages.

Wilka T'ika, Southern Peru

This is a stunning garden lodge in the sacred valley of the Urubamba which is now used as the home base for spiritual tours of Peru. A typical day starts with a yoga session in the purpose-built yoga room, followed by an organic vegetarian buffet. You may then decide to take a soul-nourishing hike into the breathtaking surrounding countryside, before travelling to Machu Picchu, Ollyantaytampu, Cusco or the Amazon Basin. The promise here is that you will get a 'spiritual experience' rather than a photo opportunity of Peru – in other words, you'll get below the surface of this amazing country. To achieve this, in addition to the yoga and mediation practice, you will meet with Peruvian herbalists, musicians and priests. You can choose to take part in sacred Peruvian rituals and meditations and meet an authentic Amazonian shaman (traditional healer), who can share some of the secrets of journeying. The highlights of the trip, according to one reviewer, were the Ayahuasca ceremony with an Amazonian shaman and the private midnight meditation at Machu Picchu. Ayahuasca, also known as the 'little death', is the psychotropic plant the shamans use to achieve an altered state of consciousness in preparation for shamanic journeying.

Chiva Som, Thailand

This Monastic-like spa and retreat in Thailand is three hours from Bangkok. The name means 'Haven of Life'. Very expensive, there's a ratio of four members of staff to every guest. The emphasis here is on the kind of unbridled luxury that never fails to attract celebrity guests. The spa occupies a tropical garden, complete with floodlit lake, Thai pagodas, Monet-esque bridges and scattered buddhas. You are encouraged to stay put, so if your true agenda is an urge to discover the real Thailand, this is not the place for you. The reason it makes our wish list is because of the quality of the treatments, the peace and quiet and the dedication to reconnecting people to their own spiritual calling. Tai chi, beach power-walking, Thai boxing, aqua-aerobics, stretch classes, yoga, meditation, fruit carving and even lessons in healthy Thai cuisine are all on offer, plus beauty therapies, massage, a turmeric-based body scrub and a Thai mud wrap. Freespirited.com Reviewer, Emma Moore, who is the Health & Beauty Director of the *Sunday Times'* Style magazine, says: 'Blissful if you're exhausted and in need of a break, but not for the more active who might find it all a bit too monastic.' Another reviewer, the UK writer Anna Pasternak, loved it and cannot wait to go back.

Posada Del Torcal, Andalucia, Spain

Leave the sparkling Mediterannean sea to others and head into the hills near Malaga in Spain to this charming hideaway for body and soul. Run by an Englishwoman and her Finnish partner, this small Andalusian hotel is set among the almond groves and breathtaking beauty of the El Torcal National Park. Each of the eight ensuite bedrooms is named after a famous Spanish artist. There is enough floorspace in each to practise an astanga yoga series or to sit quietly in meditation. In fact, the quiet ambience of the hotel makes it a favourite with those of us who have stumbled across it, usually by word-of-mouth. It is hard not to feel better when you dine alfresco on the spacious terrace with its stunning views across the valley. You can swim at the hotel's own pool – and swimming is one of the best ways into a deep meditation – or ride at nearby stables, but to reconnect with a sense of your own soul and to reflect on the beauty and sacredness of the natural world, climb to the top of the Torcal, find a warm rock and sit quietly in the sun. The shamans are always initiated into their healing path with a vision quest, which involves leaving the safety of their own hearth to spend a few days out in the wilds. There, they will be sent messages from the ancestor spirits. A hawk flying overhead or a snake coiling up behind a nearby rock may be symbolic. Whatever animal comes will have a message for the would-be shamanic healer. You may feel too faint-hearted and even afraid of being alone in wide open spaces to risk anything so challenging but a few hours in this wild and unspoiled location will soon have you plugged back in.

You can see a photograph of this stunning hideaway by logging onto the Internet and searching the name via one of the search engines such as Lycos.

St Katherine's, Parmoor, UK

If you are looking for spiritual rejuvenation in a rural idyll, this quiet and historic retreat house in Parmoor, Oxfordshire will help you put a new perspective on your life's journey. Standing in 12 acres of glorious Chilterns' countryside, the front lawn boasts a magnificent cedar tree which is reputed to have grown from a seed brought back from the Lebanon by the Crusaders. The house is believed to have been owned by the Knights Templar in the 14th century, but is now home to The Community of St Katherine of Alexandria, who moved here in 1947 after being bombed out of their premises in London's Fulham. Today, St Katherine's belongs to the Sue Ryder charity, best known for its palliative care and hospice work with the terminally ill. I like this place because as soon as you step through the door, you feel enveloped by the kind of peace you cannot get in the outside world. The hushed atmosphere does not make you feel uncomfortable but quiet, which is, of course, the whole point of being here. I was introduced to St Katherine's during an intensive two-day meditation retreat, but you can come here just to be. There is a huge walled garden with magnificent scenic views, and even a small animal sanctuary with goats, geese and chickens. (As this book goes to press, the nuns are hoping for a pig to add to their menagerie!) You can sit quietly among the graves of the priests and nuns who worked and made their home here, or just lose yourself in a walk through the neighbouring countryside. The vegetarian food is plain but delicious and there is a well-stocked library if you feel the need to lose yourself in fine literature. If you have been stuck in London all week and feel a need to escape, St Katherine's – only an hour away by road – feels for all the world like a different planet.

The Practice, Leicestershire, UK

Modelled on Depak Chopra's healing centre in La Jolla, the treatments at this Leicestershire retreat are just as expensive but the overall package is cheaper for those of us based in the UK since we don't have to fly to California to experience them. Described as a place of transformation, The Practice is the brainchild of British homoeopath and Ayurvedic specialist, Jo Pickering, who set up this intimate healing and detoxification retreat to bring the ancient Indian science of life to a Western clientele. There are never more than four people staying here at any one time; if you're one of them you should, even after just two days, leave feeling more blissed out and healthier than you would after two weeks in other places. This is because the commitment to healing, rest and relaxation at The Practice is second to none. Treatments take place in the converted barn close to the 17th-century manor house that is Jo's home. The full range of traditional

Ayurvedic cleansing and detoxifying therapies includes Abhyanga – a unique herbalised oil massage which is carried out by two therapists working synchronistically to boost immunity, release toxins and relax the mind and body – and the soothing Shirodhara, where warm oil is poured in a gentle stream over your forehead to encourage profound relaxation. The accommondation is nowhere near deluxe, nor is any money spent on frills. At £500 or more for a weekend, this may seem an expensive Time Out option for most pockets, but the therapists are very serious about their healing role and the treatments are fantastic.

Swimming with Dolphins

Show me a wish-list that doesn't include this one and I'll show you someone who is probably still fast asleep, spiritually speaking!

And Finally ... Floatation ...
The Ultimate Time Out Experience
and All for the Price of a Good Lunch!

For some people (including me) this treatment marks the end of the long search.
You can meditate for hours to reach the same state of consciousness that just an
hour in a float tank will achieve. One hour of floating is said to be the equivalent
of six hours of deep, restful sleep, and you will emerge with your brain flooded
with endorphins – the mood-enhancing brain chemicals that give you a real lift.

Some float devotees say this is the closest thing to going back into the womb,
but the reason most of us try it is the promise of one blissful hour of
uninterrupted peace. The first time I tried a floatation session, I had booked it
between an interview with a Professor of Food Science and a two-hour yoga
class. I was tired and stressed thanks to a difficult cross-country drive to get
there, and late for my date with the fibreglass tank. Half an hour later, floating
in the dark, I had no idea where or even who I was.

I had wanted to try a floatation session for several months but a childhood fear of confined spaces plus an irrational idea that it might be like being sealed in a coffin had put me off. Thankfully, the first time I decided to take the plunge I was shown a tank that looked light and airy and was nothing like the heavier, more intimidating ones I had previously inspected at various health clubs before bottling out. On arrival, I was given a list of guidelines for first-time floaters and shown through to the tank room.

Although you only float for an hour, you are allocated an additional 10 minutes each side of the float for changing and showering. You shower both before getting into the tank and afterwards. There is a light inside the tank which you can keep on or switch off so, although the main light in the outside room is dimmed and eventually turned off, you do not have to float in the dark unless you choose to.

There is also an alarm button, which is reassuring, and you are handed ear plugs because the whole idea of floating is to cut out any external stimulation, including sight and sound. There is a small jar of vaseline to smear over any cuts or scratches, which would otherwise sting in the salty water and you can, again if you choose, use an inflatable neck cushion – although to release the muscles in the shoulders and neck fully it is better to float freely with your elbows and arms bent upwards, palms facing the ceiling and at shoulder level.

I have floated in the Dead Sea in Israel, but I can report that floating in total isolation in a darkened fibreglass tank is infinitely preferable. I also, the first time, made some mistakes – and survived them – which meant the second, third and fourth floats would not be as nerve-wracking. My first error was to switch the tank light off before doing a real acclimatisation with my hands. This meant that when I did want to put the light back on and open the lid, I could not find it.

The panic was momentary and not enough to put me off the benefits of floating. For one thing, the tank is not large enough for you to float too far in any direction. You cannot, for example, do a 180-degree turn. However, I was disorientated and had not factored in that I might have floated off-centre. Instead of becoming hysterical, I reasoned that since there were only four sides, all I had to do was find the one with the push-up lid attached and that was it. I opened the lid, found the light and calmed down again. Problem solved.

I mention this not to put anyone off floating but to alert first-timers to the sense of using the first float session simply to get used to the idea – and the sensation of being completely weightless – and to become familar with the tank in which you plan to float because, once you do trust that you are safe, the sensation is fantastic.

Lying in the dark listening only to the sound of my own heart gently beating, I realised I could not tell where the water ended and my body began. Actually, it didn't matter. I spent several minutes just enjoying the sensation of floating – pushing off against the sides, stretching my arms over my head – and then settled down to concentrate, meditation-style, on my breathing. There is plenty of space above you so you do not feel hemmed in, and since the tank I floated in was made of fibreglass, I did not find it threatening. When I stepped out, I felt calm, quiet and brimming with well-being.

There is an American floatation equipment business called the Samadhi Tank Company. *Samadhi* is an ancient Indian Sanskrit word familiar to all those who meditate or practise yoga. It means, loosely, a state of bliss, which is what most floaters report feeling once they settle into the environment.

The evening after my first float, I went to a yoga class where I found, instead of feeling tired, heavy and stiff, my limbs seemed, literally, to float by themselves into the various asanas. My float had also temporarily alleviated a nagging lower back pain which I had been ignoring for two months. Although this pain had not stopped me from functioning, it was still a relief to realise, for a while, it was gone.

The benefits of floating are well documented. The combination of being weightless and having no external stimuli encourages the body to relax deeply. Like meditation, it slows down the brainwaves and stimulates the production of mood-boosting endorphins, which is why you will feel so good when you step out of the tank.

Floating is used by top sportsmen and -women to accelerate recovery after strenuous exercise – there are wonderful anecdotes about second-rate US baseball teams acquiring floatation tanks and soaring straight to the top of the league – and it is even said to rebalance the left and right sides of the brain so that you may get your most creative insights not during a brainstorming business meeting but while silently blissing out in a tank of warm, salty water.

The salt used is Epsom salts. There are 320kg added to every 775 litres of water, giving it a soft, silky feel. The water, which is just 25cm (10in) deep, is kept at skin temperature. This is why it can be hard to feel where it starts and you stop. The addition of the Epsom salts, which are used in natural healing to encourage detoxification, means that as well as being an excellent anti-stress tool, a float can also improve the condition of your skin.

Epsom salts, which are mostly magnesium sulphate, are so effective at lowering blood pressure that in a recent US study, scientists found that pregnant women suffering from high blood pressure caused by pre-eclampsia did much better when treated with Epsom salts than when anticonvulsant drugs were used.

We have an American scientist to thank for the floatation tank. Dr John Lilly was working with the US National Institute of Mental Health when he first devised an isolation chamber in the early 1950s and found himself a champion of the benefits of floating. He was investigating what happens to the brain when all external stimuli are switched off. The theory, before his work, was that the brain would shut down and drift off into a coma-like, dreamless sleep. Lilly was able to show that this was not true and that the brain carries on progamming, creating its own input, sifting information and working but in a more creative way: 'I found the tank was and is a rich and vast source of new experience. One is not deprived, one is rewarded,' he reported.

Which is, of course, exactly what you want and need from whatever way you choose of taking Time Out for yourself.

Enjoy the journey!

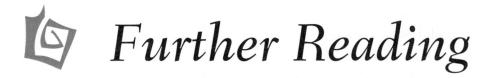

Further Reading

More about Spa Breaks and Holistic Holidays

Fodor's Healthy Escapes (Fodor Travel Publications Inc.)
Healthy Breaks in Britain & Ireland by Catherine Beattie (Discovery Books)
101 Vacations to Change Your Life by Karin Baji Holms (Citadel Press)
SpaFinder's Guide to Spa Vacations at Home and Abroad by Jeffrey Joseph (Wiley)
Vacations That Can Change Your Life by Ellen Lederman (Source Books)

Staying Healthy When You Get Home

Beat Stress and Fatigue by Patrick Holford (Piatkus)
Boost Your Immune System by Jennifer Meek and Patrick Holford (Piatkus)

The Creation of Health by Caroline Myss & C. Norman Shealy, MD (Bantam
  Books)
The 5 Laws For Healthy Living by Angela Hicks (Thorsons)
Food Combining For Health by Doris Grant & Jean Joice (Thorsons)
Maryon Stewart's Zest for Life Plan (Headline)
Vitamin Diet by Angelika Ilies (Gaia Books)

Energy and Well-Being

The Body Shop Book of Wellbeing (Ebury Press)
The Book of Energy by Cynthia Blanche (Time Life Books)
Energy Drinks by Friedrich Bohlmann (Gaia Books)
The Illustrated Encyclopedia of Well Being edited by Dr Julian Jessel-Kenyon;
  consultant editor, C. Norman Shealy (Godsfield Press)
Increase Your Energy by Louis Proto (Piatkus)

Relaxation Skills

Anti Stress by Dagmar von Cramm (Gaia Books)
The Book of Calm by Fiona Toy (Time Life Books)
Easy Exercises to Relieve Stress by Hussein Eshref (Frances Lincoln)
Healing Relaxation by Eddie Irwin (Random House)

Beauty and Well-being

The Beauty Bible by Sarah Stacey & Josephine Fairley (Kyle Cathie Ltd)
Beauty and the East – A Book Of Oriental Bodycare by Wendy Buonaventura
   (Saqi Books)
Beauty Wisdom by Bharti Vyas with Claire Haggard (Thorsons)

DeToxing

Cleanse Your System by Amanda Ursell (Thorsons)
Detox by Angelika Ilies (Gaia Books)
DETOX Your Life by Jane Scrivner (Piatkus)
Eating with the Seasons by Paula Bartimeus (Element)
The Food Combining 2-Day Detox by Kathryn Marsden (Pan Books)
Food Science, Nutrition & Health by Brian A. Fox & Allan G. Cameron (Arnold)

Ayurvedic Medicine

The Book of Ayurveda by Judith H. Morrison (Gaia Books)
The Complete Book of Ayurvedic Home Remedies by Vasant Lad (Piatkus)
The Complete Illustrated Guide to Ayurveda by Gopi Warrier & Deepika
   Gunawant (Element)
Healing With Ayurveda by Angela Hope-Murray and Tony Pickup (Gill &
   Macmillan)

Yoga and Meditation

The Complete Idiot's Guide to Meditation by Joan Budilovsky & Eve Adamson (Alpha Books)

The Complete Idiot's Guide to Power Yoga by Geo Takoma (Alpha Books)

Healing with Meditation by Doriel Hall (Gill & Macmillan)

Insight Meditation by Jack Goldstein (Newleaf)

A Little Light on Yoga by B.K.S. Iyengar (Schocken Books)

Principles of Meditation by Christina Feldman (Thorsons)

Teach Yourself Yoga by Mary Stewart (Hodder & Stoughton)

Yoga Made Easy by Demond Dunne (Prentice-Hall Inc)

Bibliography

Animal-Speak by Ted Andrews (Llewelyn Publications, 1998)

Animal-Wise by Ted Andrews (Llewelyn Publications, 1999)

Beat Eczema and Psoriasis by Stephen Terrass (Thorsons, 1999)

The Bhagavad Gita translated and introduced by Eknath Easwaran (Penguin, 1985)

The Book of Herbal Wisdom by Matthew Wood (North Atlantic Books, 1997)

Botanical Influences on Illness by Melvyn R. Werbach M.D. and Michael T. Murray N.D. (Third Line Press, 1994)

Breathe Free – Nutritional and Herbal Care for your Respiratory System by Daniel Gagnon and Amadea Morningstar (Lotus Press, 1995)

The Clinician's Handbook of Natural Healing by Gary Null, PhD. (Kensington Books, 1997)

The Complete Woman's Herbal by Anne McIntyre (Gaia Books, 1994)

Dictionary of Alternative Medicine by Joseph C. Segen M.D. (Appleton & Lange, 1998)

Don't Drink the Water by Lono Kahuna Kupua A'O (Kali Press, 1996)

Eating with the Seasons by Paula Bartimeus (Element, 1998)

Encyclopedia of Natural Medicine (revised 2nd edition) by Michael Murray N.D. and Joseph Pizzorno, N.D. (Prima Health, 1998)

The Encyclopedia of Natural Remedies by Louise Tenney M.H. (Woodland Publishing Inc. 1995)

Enzyme Potentiated Desensitization by Dr L. M. McEwen (1993; available from his clinic, see Resources)

Everything Starts from Prayer by Mother Teresa (White Cloud Press, 1998)

The Family Guide to Homeopathy by Dr Andrew Lockie (Hamish Hamilton Ltd, revised 1998)

The Food Medicine Bible by Earl Mindell (Souvenir Press, 1994)

H_2O – Healing Water for Mind and Body by Anna Selby (Collins & Brown, 2000)

Healing Drinks by Anne McIntyre (Gaia Books, 2000)

The Healing Energies of Water by Charlie Ryrie (Gaia Books, 1999)

The Healing Sun by Richard Hobday (Findhorn Press, 1999)

Healing with Whole Foods by Paul Pitchford (North Atlantic Books, 1993 revised)

Heinerman's Encyclopedia of Nuts, Berries and Seeds by John Heinerman (Parker Publishing Company, 1995)

Herb Craft – A Guide to the Shamanic and Ritual Use of Herbs by Susan Lavendar and Anna Franklin (Capall Bann Publishing, 1996)

Light on Yoga by B. K. Iyengar

A Modern Herbal by Mrs M. Grieve F.R.H.S. (Tiger Books, first published 1931; revised edition published 1994)

Natural Health Secrets from Around the World edited by Glenn W. Geelhoed M.D. and Jean Barilla M.S. (Keats Publishing, 1995)

Natural Medicine – A Practical Guide to Family Health by Beth Maceoin (Bloomsbury, 1999)

The Natural Pharmacy by Schuyler W. Lininger, Jr, D.C., Alan R. Gaby M.D., Steve Austin N.D., Donald J. Brown N.D., Jonathan V. Wright M.D., Alice Duncan D.C., C.C.H., (2nd edition), (Prima Publishing, 1999)

Not Milk … Nut Milks by Candida Lea Cole (Woodbridge Press, 1997)

Plant Spirit Medicine by Eliot Cowan (Swan Raven & Co, 1995)

The Professional's Handbook of Complementary and Alternative Medicines by Charles W. Fetrow, PharmD and Juan R. Avila, PharmD (Springhouse, 1999)

Nerys Purchon's Handbook of Natural Healing (Allen Unwin, 1998)

Restore Your Health – The Dead Sea Way by Sandra Gibbons (Green Library, 1994)

The Spiritual Properties of Herbs by Gurudas (Cassandra Press, 1988)

The Vitality Cookbook by Susan Clark (HarperCollins, 1999)

Water Can Undermine Your Health by N. W. Walker (Norwalk Press, edited and revised 1995)

Water – The Shocking Truth by Paul and Patricia Bragg (Health Science, 1998)

The Way of the Shaman by Michael Harner (HarperSanFrancisco, 1980, 1990)

The Which? Guide to Complementary Medicine by Barbara Rowlands (Penguin, 1997)

The Wisdom of the Christian Mystics by Timothy Freke (Godsfield, 1998)

The Yeast Syndrome by John Parks Trowbridge (Bantam Books, 1986)

Yoga Made Easy by Desmond Dunne (The Guernsey Press Co, reprinted 1999)

Your Body's Many Cries for Water by F. Batmanghelidj (Global Health Solutions Inc, 1992, 1995, 1997)

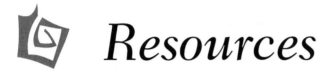 # Resources

I/BodyWorks

UK numbers are printed with the STD. For overseas, please check the correct international dialling code. Where no website address is given, none is available as this book goes to press.

Food

British Association of Nutritional Therapists
Provides a list of qualified nutritionists
0870 606 1284

The Fresh Network
UK-based subscription group providing advice and resources for a Raw Food diet
0870 800 7070
www.fresh-network.com

Institute of Optimum Nutrition
UK-based group training nutritional consultants
020 8877 9993
www.optimumnutrition.co.uk

Juice Mart Inc. (US)
++818-992-4442
www.juicemart.com

Soil Association
Champion and certifier of organic produce in the UK
0117 929 0661
www.soilassociation.org

The Vegetarian Society (UK)
0161 928 0793
www.vegsoc.org

www.veg.org
an index to links of interest to vegetarians and vegans

Air

Air Improvement Centre (UK)
020 7834 2834
www.air-improvement.co.uk

California Breath Clinics (US)
++ 323-933-7225
www.therabreath.com

Higher Nature
UK supplier for Germanium cosmetic products
01435 882880
www.highernature.co.uk

Revital
UK supplier for Oralmat supplement
0800 252875
www.revital.com

The Sivananda Yoga Centre
020 8780 0160
UK supplier of Jala Netti Pots, mats, etc.
For other countries, visit the web site:
www.sivanandayoga.org

Water

Aquathin – The PureH2O Company
UK supplier of water purification systems
01252 860111
www.pureh2o.co.uk

Aquarian Angel Services
UK supplier of water-energising devices
0700 0111811
email: mklewis@talk21.com

National Pure Water Association (UK)
01924 254433
www.hpwa.freeserve.co.uk

Sunlight

Dermalux Ltd
UK supplier of Light Boxes to treat Seasonal Affective Disorder (SAD)
020 8553 6994
www.dermalux.co.uk

Outside In
UK supplier of Light Boxes, Daylight Alarm Clocks, etc for SAD
01954 211955
www.outsidein.co.uk

Seasonal Affective Disorder Syndrome Association (UK)
Support and resources group
01903 814942

ShapeShifting (Exercise)

The Aquatic Exercise Association (US)
++941-486 8600
www.aeawave.com

The School of Tai Chi Chu'an (UK)
07626 914540
www.gn.apc.org/tai chi

Stephen Shaw
UK teacher of The Alexander Technique for swimming
020 8906 8118
www.art-of-swimming.com

Tai Chi UK
020 7407 4775
www.tai.chi.co.uk

II/Top-to-Toe

Acne

Acne Support Group (UK)
020 8841 4744
ww.stopspots.org

Allergy

Action Against Allergies
020 8892 2711
email: aaa@actionagainstallergy.freeserve.co.uk

American Academy of Allergy, Asthma & Immunology
++800-822-2762
www.aaaai.org

British Allergy Foundation
020 8303 8525
www.allergyfoundation.com

British Institute for Allergy & Environmental Therapy
Can provide a list of doctors who practise Enzyme Potentiated Desensitisation
(EPD) allergy treatment
01974 241376

Alternative/Complementary/Holistic Medicine

Alternative Medicine Publications (US)
www.alternativemedicicine.org

American Holistic Medical Association
++703-556-9728
www.holisticmedicine.org

Australian Alternative Health Directory
www.aahd.com.au

Australian Institute of Holistic Medicine
www.aihm.wa.edu.au

Dr Edward Bach Centre (UK)
01491 834678
www.bachcentre.com

Complementary Medical Association (UK)
020 8305 9571
www.the-cma.org.uk

Irish Association of Holistic Medicine
++-353-183-04211

School of Natural Medicine (US)
++888-593-6173
www.purehealth.com

Self Help Resource Centre (US)
++800-873-1663
www.concentric.net

Women's Health Advisory Service (Australia)
www.wa.gov.au/wac

Alzheimer's Disease

Alzheimer's Disease Society
020 7306 0606
www.alzheimers.org.uk

Amalgam Fillings

British Society for Mercury-Free Dentistry
Can arrange for toxicity testing but you pay
020 7373 3655

Dental Amalgam Mercury Syndrome (US)
++505-888-0111
www.icnr.com/uam/DAMSintro.html

Dr Jack Levenson
Holistic dentist and author
020 7370 0055
www.mercuryfree.co.uk

Arthritis

Arthritic Association (UK)
01323 639793
www.arthriticassociation.org.uk

National Arthritis and Musculoskeletal Association (UK)
++301-495-4484
www.nih.gov/niams/

Asthma

American Academy of Allergy, Asthma & Immunology
++800-822-2762
www.aaaai.org

Asthma & Allergy Foundation (US)
++800-7ASTHMA
www.aafa.org

Asthma Helpline (UK)
0345 010203

National Asthma Campaign (UK)
020 7971 0414
www.asthma.org.uk

Cancer

American Cancer Society
++800-ACS-2345
www.cancer.org

Breast Cancer Care (UK)
Helpline: 0808 800 6000
www.breastcancercare.org.uk

Bristol Cancer Help Centre
Sets the gold standard for cancer care and pioneered the holistic approach the mainstream now accepts
Helpline: 0117 980 9505
www.bristolcancerhelp.org

Cancer Alternative Information Bureau (CAIB)
Membership organisation set up by cancer survivor Tina Cooke, who organises
public conferences with the world's top cancer specialists
020 7266 1505
www.caib.co.uk

New Approaches to Cancer (UK)
Charitable support group specialising in complementary therapies
0800 389 2662
www.anac.org.uk

Nutritional Cancer Therapy Trust (UK)
01271 378809
www.webangels.co.uk/cancertherapy

People Against Cancer
Support group
++515-972-4444
www.dodgenet.com/nocancer

The Gawler Foundation
Holistic cancer support
++0359-967-1730

Chronic Fatigue

American Association of Chronic Fatigue Syndrome (US)
++206-521-1932
www.aacfs.org

Colon Health

Colonic International Association (UK)
01442 825632
www.interconnections.co.uk/health/colonic

National Association for Colitis & Crohn's Disease (UK)
01727 844296
www.nacc.org.uk

Constipation

British Digestive Disorders Foundation
www.digestivedisorders.org.uk

Dentistry

see Amalgam Fillings

Depression

Depression Alliance, UK
020 7633 9929
www.depressionalliance.org

Diabetes

The British Diabetic Association
020 7323 1531
www.diabetes.org

Diarrhoea

British Digestive Disorders Foundation
www.digestivedisorders.org.uk

Eating Disorders

Eating Disorders Association (UK)
01603 621414
www.edauk.com

Eczema

see also Supplements/Suppliers

The Alternative Centre
Holistic skin specialists treating eczema, psoriasis, etc., includes the Dead Sea
Centre, which uses Dead Sea skin treatments
020 7381 2298

National Eczema Society (UK)
Information line: 0870 2413604
www.eczema.org

Endometriosis

Endometriosis Association (Australia)
++03-9870-0536
www.endometriosis.org.au

Endometriosis Society (UK)
020 7222 2776
www.endo.org.uk

International Endometriosis Association (US)
++414-356-2200
www.endometriosisassn.org

Irish Endometriosis Association
++1-873-5702
www.endometriosis.uk

Simply Holistic Endometriosis Trust (UK)
01522 519992
www.endometriosis.co.uk

Fertility

The American Infertility Association
++516-917-3777
www.americaninfertility.org

Issue UK (National Infertility Association)
01922-722688
www.issue.co.uk

Heart Health

British Heart Foundation
020-7935-0185
www.bhf.org.uk

Centre for Nutritional Medicine
Dr Adam Carey & Co
Specialising in cardiovascular and sports health
020 7224 5053
www.2x1nutrition.com

Herbalism

American Herbalists Guild
++435-722-8434
www.healthy.net/herbalists/

American Herbal Products
++301-588-1171
www.ahpa.org

American Herb Society
www.herbsorg

British Herbal Medicine Association
01453 751389

Kitty Campion (UK)
Medical Herbalist specialising in digestive and women's disorders
020 7722 9270

General Council & Register of Consultant Herbalists (UK)
01792 655886
www.irch.org

Herb Research Foundation (US)
++303-449-2265
www.herbs.org

Herb Society of America
++440-256-0514
www.herbsociety.org

National Herbalists Association of Australia
++02-9560-7077
www.nhaa.org.au

National Institute of Medical Herbalists (UK)
01392 426022
www.btinternet.com/-nimh

Queensland Herb Society (Australia)
www.powerup.com.au/sage

Herpes

Herpes Viruses Association (UK)
020 7609 9061
www.herpes.org.uk

Homoeopathy

Ainsworths Homeopathic Pharmacy (UK)
Runs nationwide mail order service
020 7935 5330
www.ainsworths.com

American Institute of Homeopathy
++703-246-9501
www.healthy.net/aih

British Homeopathic Association
For a list of medically-qualified homeopathic practitioners
020 7935 2163

British Homeopathic Society
For a list of non-medical but qualified practitioners
01604 621400
www.homeopathy/soh.org

Irish Society of Homeopaths
++353-91-565-040
email: ishom@eirecom.net

National Centre for Homeopathy (US)
++703-548-7790
www.homeopathic.org

A. Nelson & Co. (UK)
Homoeopathic medicines
020 8780 4200
www.anelson.co.uk

The Royal London Homoeopathic Hospital (UK)
020 7837 8833

Society of Homeopaths (UK)
For non-medical but qualified practitioners
01604 621400
www.homeopathy-soh.org

IBS

IBS Network (UK)
To support those with irritable bowel syndrome (IBS)
Helpline: 0114 261 1531
www.IBSPage.com lists all links

Insomnia

American Sleep Disorder Association
++204-237-2760
www.asda.org

Australian Sleep Foundation
www.thoracic.org.au

Lupus

American Lupus Society
++886-532-2322
www.lupus.ca.org

Lupus Foundation of America Inc.
++800-558-0121
www.lupus.org

Migraines

see also Supplements/Suppliers
The Migraine Trust (UK)
020 7831 4818
www.migrainetrust.org

www.aash.org
Website to useful links for headaches and migraine

Naturopathy

American Association of Naturopathic Physicians
++206-323-7610
www.naturopathic.org/welcome.html

British College of Naturopathy & Osteopathy
020 7435 6464
www.bcno.org.uk

College of Naturopathic & Complementary Medicine
UK Training Schools
01342 410505
www.naturopathy-uk.com

General Council & Register of Naturopaths (UK)
01458 840072
www.naturopathy.org.uk

Incorporated Society of Naturopaths (UK)
0131 664 3435

Nutrition

see also Supplements/Suppliers
American Botanical Council
++512-926-4900
www.herbalgram.org

Australian Nutrition Foundation
www.nutritionaustralia.org

Centre for Nutritional Medicine
Dr Adam Carey & Co
Specialising in cardiovascular and sports health
020 7224 5053
www.2x1nutrition.com

David Crawford (UK)
Nutritionist and specialist in True Nutrition, i.e. using food and juicing, not supplements
020 8898 0670

National Nutritional Foods Association (US)
++949-622-6272
www.nnfa.org

Women's Nutritional Advisory Service (UK)
Can also advise men. Helplines charge premium rates
01273 487366
www.wnas.org.uk

Osteoporosis

National Osteoporosis Society (UK)
01761 471771
www.nos.org.uk

Pregnancy

National Childbirth Trust (UK)
0208 992 8637
www.nct-online.org

Psoriasis

see Eczema

Raynaud's Disease

Raynaud's & Scleroderma Association (UK)
01270 872776
www.raynauds.demon.uk

Skin Care

The Alternative Centre
Holistic skin specialists treating eczema, psoriasis etc.
020 7381 2298

Dr Hauschka Skincare (US)
++413-247 9907
www.hauschka.com

Helen Sher Skincare
Specialises in ranges for acne and rosacea but can be very expensive
020 7499 4022
www.sher.co.uk

Supplements/Suppliers

Ancient Formula Inc. (US)
++800-543-3026
www.feift.com/~ancient/index.html

Arthrovite
UK supplier of Glucosamine powder supplements with chondroitin and collagen
0800 0181282
www.arthrovite.com

The Back Shop (UK)
Devices and gadgets to promote back health
020 7935 9120
www.backshop.co.uk

Biocare (UK)
Mail order supplements
0121 433 8711
www.biocare.co.uk

Bioforce UK
Mail order herbal and naturopathic products
01294 277344
www.bioforce.co.uk

Bioforce US
++212-860-8358
www.biofroceusa.com

BodyWise UK
Suppliers of organic sanitaryware for women
01275 371764
www.natracare.com

Dr Christopher's Original Formulas (US)
From Sea Coast Vitamins
++800-555-6792
www.seacoastvitamins.com/christophers/christophers/html

Country Life/Dessert Essence (UK)
Manufacturer of WellMax winter supplement and pure Tea Tree oil
020 8614 1411

Ethical Nutrients (US)
From Sea Coast Vitamins
++949-368-3321
www.seacoastvitamins.com/ethicalnutrients/ethicalnutrients.html

David & Margaret Evans
Organic farmers and mail order suppliers of both SK Cream for eczema and
Mi-Gon for migraines and headaches. They work from the cow shed and there is
only one telephone line, so if you cannot get through, please be patient.
01526 832491

Farmacia
The UK's first pharmacy with on-site complementary therapies. Excellent
practitioners.
020 7831 0830
www.farmacia123.com

Farmatint (France)
Natural Hair Dyes and Colourings
++377-9350-0853

Forever Young International
Suppliers of good quality Aloe Vera juice and Living Food supplements
020 8944 5584
www.forever-young-help.com

Good Health Keeping (UK)
Membership health group providing resources, information, dietary advice and discounts on supplements.

Green Baby Co. Ltd (UK)
Everything you need from birth-toddlerhood
020 7633 5903
www.greenbaby.co.uk

Green People
Pioneering chemical-free personal and household products including the UK's first organic toothpaste
01444 401444
www.greenpeople.co.uk

Health Perceptions
Specialises in glucosamine for joint problems and launched the first 100% allicin garlic supplements
01252 861454
www.health-perception.co.uk

Higher Nature
Quality supplements and unpolluted fish oils, as well as germanium personal care products
01453 882880
www.highernature.co.uk

Holland & Barret
UK's biggest healthstore chain and supplement company
Mail order: 0800-273273

Jarrah Organic Pet Food (Netherlands)
If it has to come out of a tin, my dog won't eat anything else!
++31-341-432-623
www.jarrah.com

Jarrow Formulas Inc (US)
++310-204-6953
www.jarrowformulas.com

The Jet Lag Clinic (UK)
020 7584 9779
www.drdavidoconnell.co.uk

Jason Natural Cosmetics
Vitamin K cream for thread veins; other natural cosmetics
020 7435 5911 (UK)
http:/www.jason-natural.com

Kingfisher Natural Toothpaste (UK)
01603 630484
www.kingfishertoothpaste.com

Kombucha (US)
++818-784-2345
www.kombucha2000.com

Kombucha House, Australia
++6175-435104

Kombucha Tea Network (UK)
01225 833150
Also supplies good value Essiac herbal formula for cancer
www.kombucha.org.uk

KOSMED
Russian device to trigger the body's own healing mechanisms. Approved in the UK for pain-relief only but said to be effective against many disorders, including scarring.
0870 780554
www.kosmed.co.uk

Lichtwer Pharma (UK)
Respected supplement manufacturer. The company has invested heavily in researching a number of natural remedies, including garlic and evening primrose oil
01628 487780
www.lichtwer.co.uk

Lichtwer Pharma (US)
++732-389-9100
www.lichtwer.com

The Little Herbal Company
Herbal remedies include Themba cream for psoriasis
01484 685100
www.littleherbal.co.uk

Living Nature (UK)
Specialises in excellent organic body and skincare products, made in New Zealand
01425 477888
www.livingnature.com

Maitake Products Inc (US)
Suppliers of immune-boosting Maitake supplements
++201-229-0101
www.maitake.com

Dr Peter Mansfield
01507 601655
www.goodhealthkeeping.co.uk

Miracle Greens (US)
Supplement company
++310-207-6288
www.miracle-green.com

National Enzyme Company (US)
Enzyme supplements
++800-825-8545
www.nationalenzymecompany.com

Natural Source International Inc (US)
++562-698-8682
www.naturalsource.com

Nature's Answer (US)
Supplement company
++516-231-7492
www.naturesanswer.com

Nature's Own (UK)
Supplement company that makes alcohol-free herbal tinctures
01684 310022

Nature's Plus (US)
Supplement company
++516-293-0030
www.naturesplus.com

Naturopathic Health & Beauty Company (UK)
Also known as Blackmores
Natural cosmetics and bodycare
020 8842 3956

Neal's Yard Remedies (UK)
World-famous homoeopathic and herbal remedies
020 7371 7662
www.nealsyardremedies.com

Nelson Bach USA Ltd (US)
Homeopathic and Bach Flower Remedies
++978-988-3833
www.nelsonbach.com

New Zealand Natural Products (US)
Supplement company
++310-451-7397
www.naturallynz.com

NutriCentre (UK)
Excellent bookshop and mail order for complementary health supplies
020 7436 5122
www.nutricentre.co.uk

Omega Nutrition US Inc
Supplement company
++800-661-3529
www.omegaflo.com

Optimum Nutrition (US)
++630-236-0097
www.optimumnutr.com

Organic Consumers Association (US)
++310-399-9355
www.purefood.org

The Organic Herb Trading Company (formerly Hambleden Herbs) (UK)
Excellent organic specialist and mail order supplier
01823 401205
www.hambledenherbs.co.uk

Phytotherapy (US)
Herbal remedies
++201-891-1104

Quest Vitamins (UK)
0121 359 0056
www.questvitamins.co.uk

Rainforest Phytoceuticals (US)
++518-262-5825
www.amazonmedicines.com

Rodale Press (US)
Health publications
www.rodale.com

Revital
Top-class mail order company specialising in everything to do with complementary health. Owned by a trained pharmacist with an excellent knowledge of the products they carry and how to use them
0800 252875
www.revital.com

San Francisco Herb & Natural Food Company (US)
++800-227-2830
www.herbspicetea.com

Seeds of Change (US)
Organic foods
++323-586-4853
www.seedsofchange.com

Solgar Vitamin & Herb Company (US)
Quality supplement company
++201-678-3154
www.solgar.com

Solgar Vitamins Ltd (UK)
01442 890355
www.solgar.com

Source Naturals (US)
Supplement company, including colloidal silver
++831-461-6334
www.sourcenaturals.com

Tisserand Aromatherpy (UK)
Essential oils, etc.
01273 325666
www.tisserand.com

Toms of Maine (US)
Chemical-free toothpastes
++207-985-2944
www.toms-of-maine.com

Toms of Maine (UK)
01403 786460

III/Hands-On

Acupuncture

American Academy of Medical Acupuncture
++323-937-5514
www.medicalacupuncture.org

Australian Acupuncture Medical Association
++61-07-38-465866
www.acupuncture.org.au

British Acupuncture Council
020 8735 0400
www.acupuncture.org.uk

British Medical Acupuncture Society
01925 730727
www.medical-acupuncture.co.uk

Register of Acupuncturists (New Zealand)
++64-801-6400
www.acupuncture.co.nz

Alexander Technique

Alexander Technique International (US)
Covers all member countries
++617-497-2242
www.alextechnique.cjb.net

Australian Society for Teachers of the Alexander Technique
++1-800-339-571
www.alexandertechnique.org.au

Canadian Society for the Alexander Technique
++877-598-8897
www.canstat.ca

Society for Alexander Technique Teachers (US)
++612-824-5066
www.alexandertech.com

Society of Teachers of the Alexander Technique (UK)
020 7351 0828
www.stat.org.uk

Teachers of the Alexander Technique (US)
+800-473-0620
www.alexandertec.org

Aromatherapy

American Aromatherapy Alliance
++505-392-4005

Aromatherapy Organisations Council (UK)
020 8251 7912
www.aromatherapy-uk.org

Association of Medical Aromatherapists (UK)
0141 332 4924

International Federation of Aromatherapists (UK)
020 8742 2605
www.int-fed-aromatherapy.co.uk

National Association of Holistic Aromatherapy (US)
++415-564-6785
www.naha.org

Register of Qualified Aromatherapists (UK)
01245 227957
www.rqa-uk.org

Astanga Yoga

see Yoga

Autogenic Training

British Autogenic Association
Based at the Royal London Homeopathic Hospital
0207 713 6336
www.autogenic-therapy.org.uk

Ayurveda

Ayurvedic Company of Great Britain
020 7370 2255
www.ayurvediccompanyofgreatbritain.co.uk

Ayurvedic Institute (US)
++505-291-9698
www.ayurveda.com

Ayurvedic Medical Association (UK)
01908 617089
www.ayurvedic.co.uk

The Bowen Technique

Bowen Association (UK)
01455 841800
www.bowen-technique.co.uk

Bowen Technique America
++505-771-8000
www.usbowen.com

Bowen Technique Australia
++03-55-72-3000
www.bowtech.com

European College of Bowen Studies
01373-461873
www.thebowentechnique.com

Chakra Healing

See Healing

Chiropractice

American Chiropractic Association
++800-986-4636
www.amerchiro.org

Association of Chiropractors (New Zealand)
email: rgtaylor@clear.net.nz

British Chiropractic Association
0118 950 5950
www.chiropractic-uk.co.uk

Canadian Chiropractors' Association
++416-781-5656
www.ccachiro.org

Chiropractic Association of Ireland
++04-444-4837
email: ramercy@tinet.ie

Chiropractic Association of South Africa
www.chiropractic.co.za

Chiropractors' Association of Australia
++02-47-31-8011
www.caa.com.au

European Federation of Professional Chiropractic Associations
www.efpc.org

McTimoney Chiropractic Association (UK)
01865 880974
www.mctimoney-chiropractic.org

Cranial Osteopathy

see also Osteopathy

BioCranial Academy
++704-527-7173 (USA)
01247 463351 (UK)
http://dnausers.d-n-a.net/biocranial

Cranio-Sacral Therapy Association (UK)
01886 884121
www.craniosacral.co.uk

International Cranial Association (UK)
020 8367 5561

Crystal Therapy

Affiliation of Crystal Healing Organisations (UK)
01479 841450

International College of Healing (UK)
01227 472435
www.crystaltherapy.co.uk

Vantol College of Crystal Healing (UK)
01932 348815
www.crystalcollege.com

The Feldenkrais Method

Feldenkrais Information Centre (UK)
07000 785506
www.feldenkrais.co.uk

Flower Remedies

see also Phytobiophysics

Dr Edward Bach Centre
01491 834678
www.bachcentre.com

Dr Edward Bach Healing Society (US)
++508-988-3833

Flower Essence Fellowship (UK)
01225 872663

Flower Essence Services (US)
++530-265-0258
www.floweressence.com

Healing

Association of Professional Healers (UK)
01772 316726
email: majorie@aphhealers,freeserve.co.uk

Association of Therapeutic Healers (UK)
020 8671 5390
www.athealers.com

British Alliance of Healing Associations (UK)
01872 865827
email: celestine@compulink.co.uk

Confederation of Healing Organisations (UK)
01442 870660

National Federation of Spiritual Healers (UK)
01932 783164
www.nfsh.org.uk

Spiritualist Association of Great Britain
020 7235 3351

Spiritualists National Union (UK)
0845 4580768
www.snu.org.uk

World Federation of Spiritual Healers (UK-based)
01373 471553
www.wfh.org.uk

Hellerwork

Hellerwork International (US)
++707-441-4949
www.hellerwork.com

Herbalism

East West College of Herbalism (UK)
01342 822312
email: ewcolherb@aol.com

Hypnotherapy

American Institute of Hypnotherapy
++707-579-9023
www.sonic.net/hypno

British Hypnotherapy Association
020 7723 4443
01772 701248
www.hypnotherapy-uk.org

British Society of Medical & Dental Hypnosis
020 8905 4342
www.bsmdh.org

National Council for Hypnotherapy (UK)
01590 683770

Iridology

Guild of Naturopathic Iridologists (UK)
020 7821 0255
www.gni-international.org

Kinesiology

Association of Kinesiology in Ireland
++353-1457-1183

Association of Systematic Kinesiology (UK)
020 8399 3215
www.kinesiology.co.uk

International College of Applied Kinesiology (US)
++913-384-5336
www.icakusa.com

International Kinesiology College (Australia)
++61-07-5530-8899
www.about-australia.com/hsa/

Kinesiology Federation (UK)
0116 261 2326
www.kinesiologyfederation.org

KOSMED/SCENAR

Kosmed – Training and Practitioners (UK)
01488 684008
www.kosmed.co.uk

McTimoney

see Chiropractice

Massage

American Massage Therapy Association
++847-864-0123
www.amtamassage.org

British Federation of Massage Practitioners
01772 861063
www.jolanta.co.uk

British Massage Therapy Council
01865 774123
www.bmtc.co.uk

Holistic Massage Practitioners Association (South Africa)
021-782-5909

Massage Therapy Institute of Great Britain
020 7724 4105
www.cmhmassage.co.uk

Manual Lymphatic Drainage

Manual Lymphatic Drainage Association (UK)
01865 340385
www.mlduk.org.uk

The Metamorphic Technique

Metamorphic Association (UK)
020 8672 5971
www.metamorphic@britishisles.freeserve.co.uk

Osteopathy

American Osteopathic Association
++312-280-5800
www.aoa-net.org

Association of Medical Osteopaths (UK)
020 7262 5250

British Osteopathic Association
01582 488455
www.osteopathy.org

Canadian College of Osteopathy
++416-323-1465
www.ceo.edu/osteopathy/index.html

College of Osteopaths (UK)
020 8905 1937

General Council & Register of Osteopaths (UK)
0118 957 6585
www.osteopathy.org.uk

General Osteopathic Council (UK)
020 7357 6655
www.osteopathy.org.uk

Phytobiophysics

see also Flower Remedies

Phytobiophysics
01777 706155
www.phytobiophysics.co.uk

Pilates

Australian Pilates Method Association
++61-029-929-8807
www.bodycontrol.co.uk/australia.html

Body Control Pilates Association (UK)
0870 169 0000
www.bodycontrol.co.uk

Body Control Pilates (US)
1-800-Pilates
www.bodycontrol.co.uk/usa

Pilates Body Control (South Africa)
027-0826-872-422
www.bodycontrol.co.uk/south.africa.html

Pilates Foundation (UK)
0707 1781859
www.pilatesfoundation.com

Reflexology

Association of Reflexologists (UK)
0870 567 3320
www.reflexology.org

British Reflexology Association
01886 821207
www.britreflex.co.uk

British School of Reflexology
01279 429060
www.footflexology.com

International Federation of Reflexologists (UK)
020 8667 9458
www.reflexology-ifr.com

International Institute of Reflexology
01225 865899 (UK)
++813-343-4811 (US)
www.leuickm.freeserve.co.uk/homenew.htm

Reiki

International Centre for Reiki Therapists
++800-332-8112
www.reiki.org

Reiki Association (UK)
01584 891197
www.reikiassociation.org.uk

Rolfing

The Rolf Institute (UK)
020 7328 9026

The Rolf Institute (US)
++303-449-5903
www.rolf.org

Shiatsu

Australian Shiatsu College
++03-9534-4780
www.shiatsu.aimtec.net.au

British School of Shiatsu-do
020 7281 1412
www.shiatsuplace.com

European Shiatsu School
01672 513444
www.shiatsu.org.uk

Shiatsu Society of the UK
01788 555051
www.shiatsu.org

The Shiatsu Therapy Association of Australia
++039-752-6711
www.yogaplace.com/shiatsu/STAA/STAAframem.htm

Spiritual Healing

see Healing

Traditional Chinese Medicine (TCM)

College of Integrated Chinese Medicine
Accredited European training school
0118 950 8880
www.cicm.org.uk

Register of Chinese Herbal Medicine (UK)
020 8904 1357
www.rchm.co.uk

Yoga

American Yoga Association
++941-927-4977
http:/users.aol.com/amyogassn/

Astanga Yoga
www.yoga.co.uk

Australian Institute of Yoga and Ayurvedic Medicine
++03-9525-6901
www.hotkey.net.au

British Wheel of Yoga
01529 306851
www.bwy.org.uk

International Association of Yoga Therapists (US)
++707-928-9898
www.yrec.org/iayt.html

Iyengar Yoga Institute (UK)
020 7624 3080
www.iyi.org.uk

Yoga Biomedical Trust (UK)
020 7419 7195
www.yogatherapy.org

Zero Balancing

Zero Balancing Association (UK)
01308 420007
www.zerobalancing.com

IV/SoulWorks

Medicine Now!

British Biomagnetic Association
01803 293346
email: secretary@britishbiomagneticassoc.fsnet.co.uk

Colour and Light Therapy
www.mindbodyhealing.com
www.herbalchemy.com/colour.htm

Light Therapy for SAD
1-808-946-3185
www.maxpages.com/durotest/light-therapy-for-SAD

Morning Star Light
978 266 1500
www.morningstarlight.com

The Society for Light Treatment and Biological Rhythms
0115 924 9924 ext 42050
www.omni.ac.uk/umis/detail/C0005511.htm

Animal Magic

The Academy of Shamanic Studies New Zealand
www.shamanic.ac.nz

Eagle Wing Centre
www.shamanism.co.uk
020 7435 8174

Foundation for Shamanic Studies
www.shamanism.org
415 380 8280

Institute for Shamanic Studies
www.icss.org

Leslie Kenton
www.qed-productions.com/lkwhois.htm
email: leslie@qed-productions.com

Raven Lodge
www.shamana.co.uk

The Sacred Trust
www.sacredtrust.co.uk
email: mail@scaredtrust.co.uk

Shamanic Fellowship
530 620 8505
http://shamanic.org

Meditation and Prayer

Meditation Society of America
www.meditationsociety.com
email: medit8@meditationsociety.com

Transcendental Meditation UK
08705 413733
www.transcendental-meditation.org.uk

Transcendental Meditation US
888 532 7686
www.tm.org

World Wide Online Meditation Centre
www.meditationcentre.com
email jmalloy@meditationcentre.com

Time Out

The Institute of Yoga, (Kaivalya Dhama), Lonavala, India
tel ++410 403 02114 73001/73039
fax ++410 403 02114 71983

Galleon Beach, Antigua, West Indies
++1 268 460 1024
email galleonbeach.com

Wilka t'ika, Southern Peru
www.travelperu.com

Chiva Som, Thailand
Chiva-Som International Health Resort
73/4 Petchkasem Road
Hua Hin, Prachuab Khiri Khan 77110, Thailand
email genmgr@chivasom.co.th
tel ++66 32 536-536
fax ++66 32 511-154

Posada del Torcal, Andalucia, Southern Spain
++34 9 5 203 11 77
www.andalucia.com/posada-torcal

St Katherine's Retreat House, UK
Contact the warden in writing at: St Katherine's, Parmoor, Nr Frieth, Henley-on-Thames, Oxfordshire, RG9 6NN. Ask for details too of local teacher Nicola Temporal's two-day meditation retreats which she runs here.

The Practice, Leicestershire, UK
0116 259 6633
www.thepractice@demon.co.uk

Swimming with Dolphins
www.dolphinswim.com

Where to Float in the UK
www.cyberfloat.clara.net/5htm